rTMS Treatment for Depression

Paul B. Fitzgerald • Z. Jeff Daskalakis

rTMS Treatment for Depression

A Practical Guide

Second Edition

Springer

Paul B. Fitzgerald
Epworth Healthcare and Monash University
Epworth Centre for Innovation in
Mental Health
Camberwell, VIC, Australia

Z. Jeff Daskalakis
Department of Psychiatry
UC San Diego Health System
La Jolla, CA, USA

ISBN 978-3-030-91518-6 ISBN 978-3-030-91519-3 (eBook)
https://doi.org/10.1007/978-3-030-91519-3

This Springer imprint is published by the registered company Springer Nature Switzerland AG
The registered company address is: Gewerbestrasse 11, 6330 Cham, Switzerland

Contents

1 An Introduction to the Basic Principles of TMS and rTMS

Abstract

Transcranial magnetic stimulation (TMS) is a technique for stimulating brain activity that is dependent on several basic physical principles. When a substantial electrical current is induced in a stimulating coil, this is able to produce a transient time variable magnetic field. When a magnetic field of this sort and of sufficient strength is applied to the brain, it can induce an electrical current in the brain producing firing of groups of nerve cells. When TMS is applied repeatedly, it will progressively change brain activity. Low-frequency stimulation is able to reduce activity in underlying brain tissue, but high-frequency stimulation increases the activity. The discovery and practical application of these basic techniques has led to the widespread use of rTMS in neuroscientific and clinical applications.

1.1 Introduction

Transcranial magnetic stimulation (TMS) is a unique experimental and therapeutic tool that allows researchers to noninvasively stimulate and study the cortex in healthy and diseased states [1] (Fig. 1.1). It has been used as an investigational tool to measure a variety of cortical phenomena including cortical inhibition and plasticity [2, 3], as a probe to explore cognitive mechanisms [4], and as a treatment tool in illnesses such as depression and schizophrenia [5, 6]. This chapter will review the physical principles of TMS and repetitive and the neuronal structures activated by the techniques (Box 1.1).

P. B. Fitzgerald, Z. J. Daskalakis, *rTMS Treatment for Depression*,
https://doi.org/10.1007/978-3-030-91519-3_1

Box 1.1 A Note on Terminology

TMS refers to the general process of transcranial magnetic stimulation, using a time variable magnetic field to induce the firing of cortical neurons. This will encompass the use single or paired TMS pulses in experimental paradigms as well as other applications of the technology.

rTMS, or repetitive transcranial magnetic stimulation, refers to the application of repeated TMS pulses, usually at a set frequency, with the intention to make a transient or longer lasting change to local and potentially distributed brain activity.

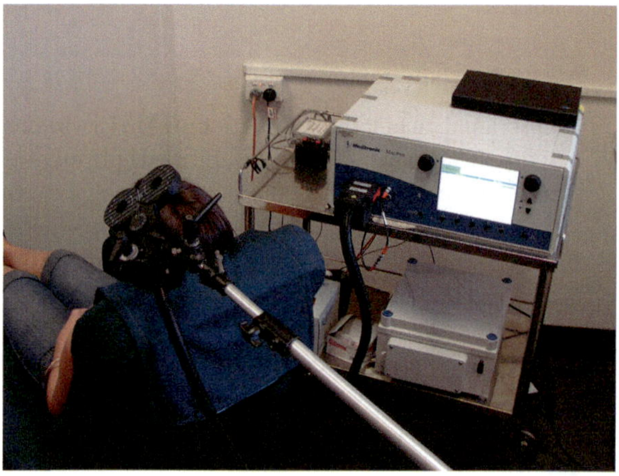

Fig. 1.1 A figure-of-eight MagVenture coil held over the head in a custom-built stand connected to a MagPro R30 device

1.2 Overview of TMS Technology

The use of TMS is dependent on some basic physical principles, first described in the nineteenth century. In 1831 Michael Faraday demonstrated that a current was induced in a secondary circuit when it was brought in close proximity to the primary circuit in which a time-varying current was flowing. Here, a changing electrical field produces a changing magnetic field that, consistent with Faraday's law, causes current to flow in a nearby conducting material. With TMS, electrical charge is stored in capacitors. Periodic discharge of this stored energy from the capacitors and through a conducting coil produces a time-varying electrical field. This electrical field produces a transient magnetic field that will cause current to flow in an appropriately located secondary conducting material, such as neurons in superficial layers of the cortex. If this current induced in the brain is of sufficient strength, it will produce depolarization of the conducting neural tissue located just under the coil.

As described electrical fields that are applied to neurons can excite these cells. The electrical field will produce a current in the intracellular and extracellular space.

This causes cell membranes to become depolarized. An action potential is initiated when this depolarization is of significant magnitude. Electrical fields experienced resistance because of scalp and skull and other intermediary tissue. Magnetic fields, by contrast, experience absolutely no resistance from the abovementioned structures. The magnetic field strength, however, is significantly reduced in relationship to the distance between the stimulating target and the magnetic source.

In regard to the generation of the TMS pulse, the requisite circuit includes a capacitor, a thyristor switch, and a coil. Charge and discharge of the capacitor are coordinated by the thyristor switch which acts as gate for conduction of the electrical field through the coil. The field that is subsequently produced is either monophasic or biphasic. This difference depends on the properties of the circuit that is used.

Commercially available stimulators produce two pulse types: a biphasic pulse or a monophasic pulse. A biphasic pulse is sinusoidal and is generally of shorter duration than a monophasic pulse, which involves a rapid rise from zero, followed by a slow decay back to zero. Monophasic pulses were typically used in the initial investigative applications of TMS, whereas biphasic pulses have been used in the vast majority of applications of rTMS as biphasic pulses can be produced more efficiently when applied repetitively at short intervals.

In commercially available stimulators, multiple types of coils are typically used. These include circular and figure-of-eight shaped coil. In general, figure-of-eight shaped coils produce a stronger and more focused magnetic field with better spatial resolution of activation compared to circular coils [7]. In contrast, circular coils tend to produce larger and deeper fields. This may be preferred when the neuroanatomic target is not precise. Iron-core coils, as used in the Neuronetics rTMS system (see Chap. 17), are advantageous in that they tend to require less power to produce strong magnetic fields and, as a corollary, generate less heat [8]. By contrast, more traditional round or figure-of-eight copper coils generate significant heat that increases as more pulses are delivered. Two methods are used to dissipate this heat. Air can be used to effectively dissipate heat and some commercially available stimulators are indeed air-cooled. One drawback to air cooling is the loud noise of the air compressor or additional weight of a fan if this is placed directly on the coil itself.

Liquid cooling can also be used. In this method the liquid helps dissipate the heat by surrounding the coil allowing for rapid heat exchange from the copper wiring to the liquid which is contiguous but not in direct contact with the coil. H-coils are a newer class of coils with multiple coil windings developed to generate greater depth of penetration (see Chap. 17). For example, while conventional figure-of-eight coils lose 50% of their magnetic field strength when the target is more than 2 cm from the stimulator, the H-coil is able to generate sufficient field strength at 6 cm [9]. This may be advantageous given the role of deeper cortical structure (e.g., the dorsal anterior cingulate and subgenual cingulate) in the pathophysiology of depression.

By and large, in small figure-of-eight shaped coil types most commonly used in rTMS treatment of depression, neurons are activated in a cortical area of approximately 2–3 cm^2 and to a depth of approximately 2 cm [10]. In most studies, figure-of-eight coils are held over the cortex flat and at about 45° from the midline position, perpendicular to the central sulcus. This induces a current from posterior to anterior direction, perpendicular to descending pyramidal neurons and parallel to interneurons, which modulate pyramidal cell firing [11]. It is the orientation between the coil and underlying neural tissue that allows researchers to selectively activate different groups of neurons providing useful information regarding neuronal inhibition, excitation, and connectivity.

1.3 Overview of Repetitive TMS (rTMS) Technology

Repetitive transcranial magnetic stimulation (rTMS) involves stimulation of the cortex by a train of magnetic pulses at frequencies between 1 and 50 Hz in contrast to single pulse TMS in which the frequency of stimulation is <1 Hz [12]. Higher frequencies can be achieved because the bipolar stimulus, as opposed to a unipolar stimulus, is shorter and requires less energy to produce neuronal excitability. Thus, capacitors can charge and discharge rapidly, thereby achieving high stimulation rates. It is the ability to achieve such high stimulation rates that has made rTMS a valuable tool in investigation and treatment of many neuropsychiatric disorders.

Repetitive TMS can either activate or inhibit cortical activity depending on stimulation frequency [13]. Low-frequency (~1 Hz) stimulation for a period of approximately 15 min induces a transient inhibition, or a decrease in activity, of the cortex [14]. The mechanisms behind such inhibition are unclear although there are similarities to long-term depression, a cellular experimental phenomena where repeated low-frequency stimulation reduces activity in individual synapses [14]. In contrast, stimulation at frequencies above 1 Hz has been shown to induce increased cortical activation [15]. The mechanisms by which such activation occurs are also unclear although some authors suggest that it may be due to a transient increase in the efficacy of excitatory synapses [16]. It has also been argued that the orientation between the coil and underlying neural tissue that allows researchers to selectively activate different groups of neurons may be key to understanding the principles mediating its therapeutic efficacy. That is, by virtue of the fact that TMS activates neurons transsynaptically [17] (i.e., activation of interneurons), neuronal stimulation can selectively activate or inhibit the cortex.

Stimulating at high frequencies has been shown to produce transient "functional" lesions in cortical areas receiving stimulation [4, 18]. Therefore, rTMS may be used as a neurophysiological probe to test the functional integrity of different cortical regions by either activating these regions or inhibiting them. It has been postulated that stimulation at high frequencies can also facilitate plasticity: the way in which the brain adapts to stimulation or environmental change. Potentiation of plasticity may also represent a mechanism through which rTMS exerts its therapeutic effects in depression. Plasticity in the cortex involves an adaptive rewiring of neurons in response to environmental change. Synaptic plasticity has long been conceptualized as a cellular substrate of learning and memory. As theorized by Hebb in 1949 [19], synaptic plasticity is represented by changes in synaptic strength in response to coincident activation of coactive cells, which manifest as long-term potentiation (LTP) or long-term depression (LTD). LTP depends, in part, on activation of a double-gated NMDA receptor that serves as a "molecular" coincidence detector.

These calcium-permeable glutamatergic receptors are able to provide a long-term augmentation of postsynaptic signal once activated by an input sufficient to depolarize postsynaptic membrane and relieve tonic Mg^{2+} inhibition [20, 21]. rTMS can cause neurons in the cortex to generate repeated and consistent firing of coactive cells, thereby producing plasticity in the cortex. Modifying plasticity has been regarded as a downstream mechanism through which serotonin reuptake inhibitors result in depression treatment [22]. rTMS therefore may exert its antidepressant effects by potentiating plasticity in the cortex.

1.4 Sham Stimulation

Double-blind placebo or sham-controlled rTMS trials are the best methods through which the clinical effects of rTMS can be optimally derived. Sham stimulation can involve lifting the coil off the person's head, thereby generating sound but no tactile sensation. It may be hard to ensure the adequacy of blinding with this form of sham control which is now rarely used. Another method through which sham rTMS can be applied is by tilting the coil at either 45° or 90° or stimulating with material between the coil and surface of the head. These methods may produce noise and some scalp sensation without generating sufficient field strength to activate the cortex. A criticism that has been levied with this approach is that the scalp sensation is very weak and, therefore, also easy to differentiate from active TMS despite the fact that subjects who participate in these trials are, for the most part, rTMS naïve. George et al. [23] reported on a novel and very effective method to which to generate sham stimulation. In this method, "active" sham stimulation is produced through an electrical field being generated by a peripheral nerve stimulator to produce scalp sensation at the stimulation site. Through these methods, the ability to predict active versus sham stimulation was reduced to chance [23].

1.5 Noise

A loud clicking noise is heard when the stimulator is discharged. This clicking noise is generated by internal stress that is caused by the rapid alternating electrical field that is produced in the capacitor, cables, and the stimulating coil. The clicking sound that is generated is between 120 and 300 dB. As such, it is always advised that both operators and subjects wear hearing projection throughout the treatment.

References

1. Barker AT, Jalinous R, Freeston IL (1985) Non-invasive magnetic stimulation of human motor cortex. Lancet 1(8437):1106–1107. Epub 1985/05/11
2. Kujirai T, Caramia MD, Rothwell JC, Day BL, Thompson PD, Ferbert A et al (1993) Corticocortical inhibition in human motor cortex. J Physiol Lond 471:501–519
3. Classen J, Liepert J, Wise SP, Hallett M, Cohen LG (1998) Rapid plasticity of human cortical movement representation induced by practice. J Neurophysiol 79(2):1117–1123

4. Flitman SS, Grafman J, Wassermann EM, Cooper V, O'Grady J, Pascual-Leone A et al (1998) Linguistic processing during repetitive transcranial magnetic stimulation. Neurology 50(1):175–181
5. Pascual-Leone A, Rubio B, Pallardo F, Catala MD (1996) Rapid-rate transcranial magnetic stimulation of left dorsolateral prefrontal cortex in drug-resistant depression. Lancet 348(9022):233–237
6. Hoffman RE, Boutros NN, Hu S, Berman RM, Krystal JH, Charney DS (2000) Transcranial magnetic stimulation and auditory hallucinations in schizophrenia. Lancet 355(9209):1073–1075
7. Ueno S, Tashiro T, Harada K (1988) Localized stimulation of neural tissue in the brain by means of a paired configuration of time-varying magnetic fields. J Appl Phys 64:5862–5864
8. Epstein CM, Davey KR (2002) Iron-core coils for transcranial magnetic stimulation. J Clin Neurophysiol 19(4):376–381. Epub 2002/11/19
9. Roth Y, Amir A, Levkovitz Y, Zangen A (2007) Three-dimensional distribution of the electric field induced in the brain by transcranial magnetic stimulation using figure-8 and deep H-coils. J Clin Neurophysiol 24(1):31–38. Epub 2007/02/06
10. Barker AT (1999) The history and basic principles of magnetic nerve stimulation. Electroencephalogr Clin Neurophysiol Suppl 51:3–21
11. Amassian VE, Deletis V (1999) Relationships between animal and human corticospinal responses. Electroencephalogr Clin Neurophysiol Suppl 51(3):79–92
12. Wassermann EM (1998) Risk and safety of repetitive transcranial magnetic stimulation: report and suggested guidelines from the International Workshop on the Safety of Repetitive Transcranial Magnetic Stimulation, June 5–7, 1996. Electroencephalogr Clin Neurophysiol 108(1):1–16
13. Fitzgerald PB, Fountain S, Daskalakis ZJ (2006) A comprehensive review of the effects of rTMS on motor cortical excitability and inhibition. Clin Neurophysiol 117(12):2584–2596
14. Chen R, Classen J, Gerloff C, Celnik P, Wassermann EM, Hallett M et al (1997) Depression of motor cortex excitability by low-frequency transcranial magnetic stimulation. Neurology 48(5):1398–1403
15. Siebner HR, Peller M, Willoch F, Minoshima S, Boecker H, Auer C et al (2000) Lasting cortical activation after repetitive TMS of the motor cortex: a glucose metabolic study. Neurology 54(4):956–963
16. Pascual-Leone A, Valls-Sole J, Wassermann EM, Hallett M (1994) Responses to rapid-rate transcranial magnetic stimulation of the human motor cortex. Brain 117(Pt 4):847–858
17. Rothwell JC (1997) Techniques and mechanisms of action of transcranial stimulation of the human motor cortex. J Neurosci Methods 74(2):113–122
18. Pascual-Leone A, Gates JR, Dhuna A (1991) Induction of speech arrest and counting errors with rapid-rate transcranial magnetic stimulation. Neurology 41(5):697–702
19. Hebb DO (1949) The organization of behavior. A neuropsychological theory. Wiley, New York
20. Bliss TV, Collingridge GL (1993) A synaptic model of memory: long-term potentiation in the hippocampus. Nature 361(6407):31–39
21. Rison RA, Stanton PK (1995) Long-term potentiation and N-methyl-D-aspartate receptors: foundations of memory and neurologic disease? Neurosci Biobehav Rev 19(4):533–552
22. Branchi I (2011) The double edged sword of neural plasticity: increasing serotonin levels leads to both greater vulnerability to depression and improved capacity to recover. Psychoneuroendocrinology 36(3):339–351. Epub 2010/09/30
23. George MS, Lisanby SH, Avery D, McDonald WM, Durkalski V, Pavlicova M et al (2010) Daily left prefrontal transcranial magnetic stimulation therapy for major depressive disorder: a sham-controlled randomized trial. Arch Gen Psychiatry 67(5):507–516. Epub 2010/05/05

The History of TMS and rTMS Treatment of Depression

2

Abstract

The use of electrical and magnetic devices to alter brain activity has been periodically suggested for many years. The actual concept of transcranial magnetic stimulation (TMS) was proposed in the late 1900s, but technology did not exist at that time to produce sufficiently strong magnetic fields to stimulate brain activity. This technology, first developed in the 1980s, is now widely used in TMS and *repetitive* transcranial magnetic stimulation (rTMS) applications including in the treatment of depression. rTMS refers to the use of repeated TMS pulses, at a specific frequency, usually with an intent to change brain activity, rather than just to produce a response to a single pulse. Initial studies investigating the capacity of rTMS to modify mood were conducted in the early to mid-1990s. Modern applications of rTMS were first enacted in studies when high-frequency rTMS was applied to the left DLPFC with these studies published in 1995 and 1996. Since that time, the field has progressed substantially with a large body of research establishing the use of rTMS and many studies exploring alternative methods of application.

2.1 Introduction

The application of electricity and magnetic fields in medicine has a long but not always distinguished history. Reports of the use of electrical techniques in medicine date back at least to the Roman Empire where in 46 AD Scribonius Largus, physician of the emperor Tiberius, described the use of torpedoes (aquatic animals capable of electrical discharge) for medical applications [1, 2].

P. B. Fitzgerald, Z. J. Daskalakis, *rTMS Treatment for Depression*,
https://doi.org/10.1007/978-3-030-91519-3_2

> *The live black torpedo when applied to the painful area relieves and permanently cures some chronic and intolerable protracted headaches ... carries off pain of arthritis ... and eases other chronic pains of the body.*
>
> *For any type of gout a live black torpedo should, when the pain begins, be placed under the feet. The patient must stand on a moist shore washed by the sea and he should stay like this until his whole foot and leg up to the knee is numb. This takes away present pain and prevents pain from coming on if it has not already arisen. In this way Anteros, a freedman of Tiberius, was cured.* (Compositiones Medicae, 46 AD)

The notion that electricity could be used for therapeutic purposes was carried through the Middle Ages and during the Renaissance gained particular attraction. In the 1600s in England, William Gilbert, physician to Queen Elizabeth, published *De Magnete*, in which he described the use of electricity in medicine. Gilbert described that when certain materials are rubbed, they will attract light objects. He coined the name "electricity" from the Greek "electron" for amber [3].

During the 1700s the use of electricity for the treatment of paralysis was suggested by Krueger, a Professor of Medicine in Germany, and Kratzenstein published a book on electrotherapy. Kratzenstein described a method of treatment which consists of seating the patient on a wooden stool, electrifying him by means of a large revolving frictional glass globe, and then drawing sparks from him through the affected body parts.

The development of the field diverged in several significant directions in the coming centuries, in parallel with the expansion of knowledge in the physical sciences. These will be briefly described in turn.

First, heralding the development of the science of electrophysiology, in 1780 in Italy, Luigi Galvani, Professor of Anatomy at the University of Bologna, first observed the twitching of muscles under the influence of electricity (prepared from the leg of a frog) [4]. Alessandro Volta subsequently demonstrated that the "galvanic" effect did not require contact with the animal (and also contributed to the development of the battery) [4]. Another Italian, Carlo Matteucci, was able to show that injured tissue generates electric current [4].

During the same time the notion of magnetism, in particular that of "animal magnetism," became widely known due to the work of Anton Mesmer. The concept was first described by Paracelsus (1530) but considerably popularized by Mesmer through his various works including the *Propositions Concerning Animal Magnetism* in 1779 and his doctoral thesis 'De influxu planetarum in corpus humanum' produced in 1766 [4]. Mesmer's concept, however, is related to magnetic properties only by analogy as he described the response of the human body to heavenly bodies and the bodies' reciprocal interaction with the environment as analogous with the properties of a physical magnet. Mesmer initially constructed physical apparatus (the *baquet*) that was used to effect the animal magnetism of a subject but latter disposed of the use of metallic objects altogether. Mesmer's ideas became very popular in certain European countries (especially Germany, Russia, and Denmark) but were progressively discredited, and Mesmer eventually closed his Paris clinic. Although Mesmer's ideas were widely disproved, especially through a series of scientific commissions in Paris, the notion that imagination (rather than magnetism) could have physical effects took hold and substantially contributed to the development of the field of hypnosis [4].

In a different direction, the notion of "magnet therapy" became widely popular through several centuries. This was based upon the presumption that electrical or magnetic stimulation could be a "nutrient" to the body that was thought of as electric. Examples of this movement include the establishment of an "electrical therapy" department which was established in the mid-1880s at Guy's Hospital in London under Dr. Golding Bird. Various "therapeutic" devices, including "electrical belts," were widely popular through the early part of the twentieth century.

2.2 Early Attempts to Develop TMS-Like Approaches

The modern concept of TMS could not be envisioned prior to the early 1800s due to lack of knowledge until that time of the properties of magnetic fields and their relationship to electrical currents. It was Michael Faraday who first outlined the principle of mutual induction in 1831 (e.g., as later described in his *Lectures on the Forces of Matter*, given at The Royal Institution of Great Britain, December 1859) [5]. This principle states that a current can be induced in a secondary circuit when its relationship to a primary circuit is altered in several specific ways, including that the primary current is turned on or off or the primary current is moved relative to the secondary current. Faraday described that this effect was mediated through the magnetic flux created by the changing circuit and that alterations in the magnetic flux would induce an electrical field [5]. The line integral of this electric field is referred to as the electromotive force and this force is responsible for the induced current flow. The magnitude of this effect can be quantified and mathematically described. Importantly, the magnitude of the force is proportional to the rate of change in the magnetic flux.

Nikola Tesla in the USA in the latter part of the nineteenth century was experimenting with the physiological effects of high-frequency currents [5]. He constructed a variety of flat-, cone-, and helix-shaped coils that were used to produce physiological effects. Tesla coils or Oudin resonators consisted of primary and secondary large coils used to produce an ionization of the air between the coils. A patient would sit between the coils and experience a sensation described by Tesla as like the "bombardment of miniature hail stones." These coils formed the basis for the latter development of diathermy that was propagated by Tesla and the Frenchman d'Arsonval. Tesla also contributed significantly to the development of X-ray [5].

D'Arsonval was also the first person to develop ideas that could be considered equivalent to modern TMS technology. He reported the effects of cranial stimulation with a large magnetic coil producing a 110 V current at 42 Hz. The coils utilized by d'Arsonval were similar to those developed by Tesla but without the secondary coil [4]. He described numerous physiological responses to his coil including the development of dilation of blood vessels, vertigo, syncope, and phosphenes. Phosphenes, or visual flashes of light, are produced with modern TMS stimulation of the occipital visual cortex, and it is possible that this was the source of the experiences produced in the experiments of D'Arsonval, although from knowledge of the capacity of technology of the day it seems more likely that they were the result of direct retinal stimulation.

As these reports were published in French, they were not widely read in the English- and German-speaking scientific communities. Independent reports of a similar nature were made by Beer in 1902 [6], and a device designed for use in the treatment of depression and other neuroses was actually patented by Pollacsek and Beer in Vienna. Widespread use of this device did not follow and one can reasonably assume that the induced fields would have been insufficient to have likely therapeutic effects. The report of Beer inspired several other investigators. Thompson produced a large 32 turn coil in which a subject's head was to be placed which produced some sight and taste sensations [7]. Dunlap reported a controlled experiment designed to test the veracity of the reports of the sensations produced with these devices "controlling" for the noise produced [8]. Visual sensations were associated with the alternating current but he was unable to confirm other sensations. Magnusson and Stevens produced two elliptical coils, which were used to produce visual sensations including flickering and a luminous horizontal bar [9].

For several decades after, little research was published in this area. In 1947 Barlow described the use of a small coil to produce visual sensations through stimulation at the temple but not the occiput. The conclusion was drawn that the site of this stimulation was retinal [10].

The field of magnetic stimulation of brain tissue did not significantly advance for the greater part of the twentieth century. Through this time, variations on electrical therapies continued to remain popular. For example, Lakhovsky working in Paris in the 1920s developed his "multiple wave oscillator," a device designed to produce a broad-spectrum electromagnetic field between two large circular electrodes [11]. The patient would sit between two of these coils and have disturbances of cellular function corrected. The therapeutic properties of devices generating fields of this type have not been established although this marginal field of medicine still has its proponents to this day. In recent years there has been a resurgence of interest in the role of pulsed weak electromagnetic fields in the treatment of disease states including multiple sclerosis, although controlled trials are lacking [12].

The direct electrical stimulation of the unexposed cortex was first attempted in the 1950s [13] but this proved too painful for its routine use. The field was further developed in the early 1980s with attempts to alter the electrical stimulation to enhance the effect and lessen discomfort, but additional problems with painful jaw contraction were encountered [14, 15]. Electrical stimulation has gained some use in experimental electrophysiology but has been largely, but not completely [16], replaced by magnetic stimulation.

2.3 The Development of Modern TMS

Modern TMS has a relatively brief history. Barker first started investigating the use of short pulsed magnetic fields to stimulate human peripheral nerves in the 1970s [17]. The first device capable of generating cortical activity was developed by Barker and others in Sheffield, England, and first described in 1985 [18]. Stimulators first attracted the attention of neurologists and neurophysiologists due to their capacity to be applied in the testing of nerve activity from the cortex to the periphery. The first therapeutic reports of the use of TMS were in the treatment of mood disorders, which emerged around the same time as reports of the capacity of TMS to alter the mood of healthy control subjects. The initial studies in healthy controls suggested that rTMS applied to the left dorsolateral prefrontal cortex (DLPFC) could induce a mild increase in self-reported sadness. rTMS applied to the right DLPFC could improve self-rated positive mood [19, 20]. Mood effects across these and other studies were relatively inconsistent and produced with differing TMS parameters. Later studies did not necessarily confirm that mood changes could be produce reliably in healthy control subjects. However, initial studies in depressed patients were also being undertaken around the same time. The very first studies utilized stimulation over the vertex and in general reported inconclusive results, especially as they were usually open-label studies in small samples [21–23]. In 1994 it was proposed that the prefrontal cortex (PFC) might be a more effective target for TMS [24]. This idea was based upon the evidence of a link between the response to electroconvulsive therapy (ECT) and changes in PFC function [25] as well as imaging studies reporting abnormalities in the PFC in depressed patients [26].

The first published studies using focal stimulation of the prefrontal context followed and appeared in 1995 and 1996. In the first of these studies, George et al. reported the treatment of six medication nonresponsive patients with 20 Hz TMS applied to the left PFC [27]. This was followed with a double-blind study of 2 weeks of treatment applied with a sham control in a crossover design [28]. Around the same time Pascual-Leone et al. reported a sham-controlled crossover study with 5 days of 10 Hz treatment [29]. The results of these two studies were sufficient to arouse the interest of researchers around the world in the use of high-frequency rTMS applied to the left DLPFC. Studies since that time have substantially extended the dose of stimulation applied, both in regard to the number of treatment sessions and to the number of pulses applied per session. However, many of the basic aspects of treatment used in these initial studies, for example, the methodology for coil placement, have not really advanced substantially since the mid-1990s. Some researchers have developed new, alternate ways to utilize rTMS. For example, Klein et al. in the late 1990s developed the approach of using low-frequency rTMS applied to the right DLPFC [30], an approach which has subsequently proven to be of similar efficacy to standard high-frequency left-sided rTMS.

References

1. Alexander FG, Selesnick S (1956) History of psychiatry. Allen and Unwin, London, p 282
2. Kirsch DL, Lerner FN (1995) Electromedicine: the other side of physiology. Chapter 23. In: Innovations in pain management: a practical guide for clinician. The textbook of the American Academy of Pain Management. GR Press, Inc, Winter Park, FL
3. Gilbert W (1600) De Magnete ("On the magnet"). Chiswick Press, London
4. Becker RO, Marino AA (1982) The origins of electrobiology. In: Becker RO, Marino AA (eds) Electromagnetism & life. State University of New York Press, Albany
5. Cheney M (1983) Tesla - man out of time. Twenty First Century Books, Breckenridge, CO
6. Beer B (1902) Ueber das Auftraten einer objective Lichtempfindung in magnetischen Felde. Klin Wochenschr 15:108–109

7. Thompson SP (1910) A physiological effect of an alternating magnetic field. Proc R Soc Lond Biol B82:396–399
8. Dunlap K (1911) Visual sensations from the alternating magnetic field. Science 33:68–71
9. Magnusson CE, Stevens HC (1911) Visual sensations caused by the changes in the strength of a magnetic field. Am J Physiol 29:124–136
10. Barlow HB, Kohn HL, Walsh EG (1947) Visual sensations aroused by magnetic fields. Am J Physiol 148:372–375
11. Lakhovsky G (1934) Apparatus with circuits oscillating under multiple wave lengths. United States Patent Office patent 1,962,565, 12 Jun 1931
12. Sandyk R (1996) Electromagnetic fields for treatment of multiple sclerosis. Int J Neurosci 87(1–2):1–4
13. Gualiterotti T, Patterson AS (1954) Electrical stimulation of the unexposed cerebral cortex. J Physiol Lond 125:278–291
14. Merton PA, Hill DK, Morton HB, Marsden CD (1982) Scope of a technique for electrical stimulation of human brain, spinal cord, and muscle. Lancet 2(8298):597–600
15. Merton PA, Morton HB (1980) Stimulation of the cerebral cortex in the intact human subject. Nature 285(5762):227
16. Rossini PM, Barker AT, Berardelli A, Caramia MD, Caruso G, Cracco RQ et al (1994) Non-invasive electrical and magnetic stimulation of the brain, spinal cord and roots: basic principles and procedures for routine clinical application. Report of an IFCN committee. Electroencephalogr Clin Neurophysiol 91(2):79–92. Epub 1994/08/01
17. Barker AT (1999) The history and basic principles of magnetic nerve stimulation. Electroencephalogr Clin Neurophysiol Suppl 51:3–21. Epub 1999/12/11
18. Barker AT, Jalinous R, Freeston IL (1985) Non-invasive magnetic stimulation of human motor cortex. Lancet 1(8437):1106–1107. Epub 1985/05/11
19. George MS, Wassermann EM, Williams WA, Steppel J, Pascual-Leone A, Basser P et al (1996) Changes in mood and hormone levels after rapid-rate transcranial magnetic stimulation (rTMS) of the prefrontal cortex. J Neuropsychiatry Clin Neurosci 8(2):172–180
20. Pascual-Leone A, Catala MD, Pascual-Leone Pascual A (1996) Lateralized effect of rapid-rate transcranial magnetic stimulation of the prefrontal cortex on mood. Neurology 46(2):499–502
21. Hoflich G, Kasper S, Hufnagel A, Ruhrmann S, Moller H-J (1993) Application of transcranial magnetic stimulation in drug-resistant major depression - a report of two cases. Hum Psychopharmacol 8:361–365
22. Kolbinger HM, Holflich G, Hufnagel A, Moller H-J, Kasper S (1995) Transcranial magnetic stimulation (TMS) in the treatment of major depression - a pilot study. Hum Psychopharmacol 10:305–310
23. Grisaru N, Yaroslavsky U, Abarbanel JM, Lamberg T, Belmaker RH (1994) Transcranial magnetic stimulation in depression and schizophrenia. Eur Neuropsychopharmacol 4:287–288
24. George MS, Wassermann EM (1994) Rapid-rate transcranial magnetic stimulation (rTMS) and ECT. Convuls Ther 10:251–253
25. Nobler MS, Sackheim H (1998) Mechanisms of action of electroconvulsive therapy. Psychiatr Ann 10:23–29
26. George MS, Ketter TA, Post RM (1994) Prefrontal cortex dysfunction in clinical depression. Depression 2:59–72
27. George MS, Wassermann EM, Williams WA et al (1995) Daily repetitive transcranial magnetic stimulation (rTMS) improves mood in depression. Neuroreport 6:1853–1856
28. George MS, Wasserman EM, Kimbrell TA, al e. (1997) Mood improvement following daily left prefrontal repetitive transcranial magnetic stimulation in patients with depression: a placebo-controlled crossover trial. Am J Psychiatry 154:1752–1756
29. Pascual-Leone A, Rubio B, Pallardo F, Catala MD (1996) Rapid-rate transcranial magnetic stimulation of the left dorsolateral prefrontal cortex in drug-resistant depression. Lancet 348:233–237
30. Klein E, Kolsky Y, Puyerovsky M, Koren D, Chistyakov A, Feinsod M (1999) Right prefrontal slow repetitive transcranial magnetic stimulation in schizophrenia: a double-blind sham-controlled pilot study. Biol Psychiatry 46(10):1451–1454

The Mechanism of Action of rTMS

3

Abstract

A considerable body of research has explored the mechanism of action of rTMS stimulation, although only some of this research is directly relevant to understanding the effects of rTMS treatment in patients with depression. High-frequency stimulation appears to produce an increase in local cortical excitability and also an alteration in the activity of local inhibitory circuits. Low-frequency stimulation produces a significant reduction in local cortical activity, although the effect of it on local inhibition is less clear. Repetitive TMS stimulation applied to prefrontal areas in patients with depression appears to alter both local cortical activity and activity in connected brain regions. This may include changes in subcortical neurotransmitter release such as with dopamine and alterations in functional and even structural connections between brain regions. Further work is required to ascertain whether the effects of rTMS occur through the induction of neuromodulatory substances such as brain-derived neurotrophic factor.

3.1 Introduction

Repetitive transcranial magnetic stimulation (rTMS) is a noninvasive method of stimulating nerve cells in cortical regions of the brain which can also produce significant therapeutic effects in a number of neurological and psychiatric disorders [1]. However, the mechanisms through which such treatment effects occur are uncertain. Generally speaking, it has been proposed that the effects of high-frequency rTMS in depression occur through an increase of activity in the left DLPFC, which is proposed to be underactive in patients with depression. Low-frequency right-sided rTMS is proposed to reduce right-sided DLPFC activity which is proposed to be overactive in patients with depression. However, rTMS has

P. B. Fitzgerald, Z. J. Daskalakis, *rTMS Treatment for Depression*,
https://doi.org/10.1007/978-3-030-91519-3_3

a complex series of effects on the brain, and research has not necessarily consistently demonstrated these relationships.

In this chapter, we will review the brain mechanisms postulated to be altered by TMS, and how they may relate to the treatment of depression.

3.2 Effects of rTMS Assessed in the Motor Cortex

The majority of research into the physiological effects of rTMS has occurred with stimulation applied to the motor cortex, where there are easily available means to study alterations in cortical activity. In particular, single and paired pulses of TMS applied to the motor cortex can be utilized to index aspects of cortical excitability and inhibition, providing a ready mechanism to study the effects of repetitive rTMS stimulation. In this regard, rTMS has been shown to result in changes in several physiological parameters in the motor cortex, including in excitability, evidenced in motor threshold (MT) and motor evoked potential (MEP) alterations; in cortical inhibition and facilitation, evidenced in silent period (SP) and paired pulse inhibition and facilitation (ppTMS) changes; and in alterations in cortical plasticity. These changes appear to be rTMS frequency and intensity dependent.

3.2.1 Effects on Motor Cortical Excitability

Low-frequency rTMS (1 Hz or less) has been shown to decrease corticospinal excitability (see review in [2]). For example, Chen et al. [3] demonstrated that a 15-min train of suprathreshold 0.9 Hz rTMS applied to the motor cortex reduced MEP size. This reduction lasted at least 15 min after the end of the stimulation train. Siebner et al. [4] found a similar reduction in MEP size in healthy controls, but not in patients with writer's cramp when 1 Hz rTMS was applied over the left primary motor hand area. These findings have been confirmed in more recent studies. Subthreshold 1 Hz stimulation for 4 [5] or 10 [6] min both resulted in significant reduction in MEP size. Muellbacher et al. [7] found that 1 Hz suprathreshold TMS for 15 min increased the motor threshold and reduced MEP amplitude. Notably, the degree of these effects has been shown to be dependent on stimulation parameters such as intensity [8].

Effects of 1 Hz stimulation may also be seen at sites not directly targeted for stimulation. Gerschlager et al. [9] used a considerably lower stimulation intensity than previous studies (90% active motor threshold (AMT) which approximately corresponds to 60–70% of resting motor threshold (RMT)). They demonstrated that prolonged 1 Hz stimulation of the premotor cortex, but not the primary motor, parietal, or prefrontal cortex, resulted in MEP suppression for at least 15 min. These authors suggest that the effects of premotor cortex stimulation are due to its rich connection to the primary motor cortex, and that such stimulation can suppress primary motor cortex excitability even more so than stimulation of the motor cortex itself. Wassermann et al. [10] found that 1 Hz rTMS reduced the excitability of the contralateral, non-stimulated motor cortex as demonstrated by a reduction in the slope of the MEP recruitment curve. Thus, low-frequency stimulation of a cortical area may evoke cortical inhibition in interconnected areas [11]. Reduction of cortical excitability with low-frequency rTMS is clearly relevant to the treatment of depression, with low-frequency stimulation evaluated as an antidepressant strategy when applied to the right DLPFC [12].

High-frequency rTMS appears most likely to have effects opposite to that of low-frequency rTMS and to result in increased motor cortical excitability when applied to the motor cortex (see [2]). For example, Pascual-Leone et al. [13] demonstrated a pattern of facilitation of MEPs produced by a train of rTMS that varied with stimulus intensity and frequency. With 5 Hz rTMS at 150% RMT, there was clear facilitation of MEPs. At 10 and 20 Hz rTMS with lower intensities (110% RMT), there was also a consistent pattern of facilitation. In contrast, with 150% RMT at 10 and 20 Hz rTMS, an alternating pattern of MEP inhibition and facilitation was demonstrated. Several other studies have also demonstrated that MEP size increases with high-frequency rTMS (>1 Hz) [14–16]. Modugno et al. [17] reported that 20 stimuli of 5, 10, and 20 Hz applied to the motor cortex at 100% RMT resulted in brief MEP suppression that lasted for about 1 s after rTMS. This suppression in the post-train interval was prolonged with longer trains or higher frequencies. Increasing the intensity of the rTMS to 130% and 150% of the RMT resulted in facilitation rather than suppression of the MEP, consistent with previous findings [15]. Therefore, high-frequency rTMS at low intensity may cause inhibition for 1–2 s after the rTMS train, whereas at higher intensity, high-frequency rTMS consistently produces facilitation. The mechanisms by which altered excitability occurs in the cortex are unclear. However, it has been suggested that decreased excitability is related to the synaptic process of long-term depression [3], whereas increased excitability has been related to long-term potentiation [18].

The relevance of these studies to understanding the mechanism of action of rTMS in depression is uncertain. Clearly, individual high-frequency rTMS trains applied to the motor cortex increase excitability. However, what is less clear is an understanding of the effects of cumulative stimulation trains over a long treatment session, and the accumulation of changes in cortical excitability with daily rTMS sessions over a matter of weeks as is applied in treatment protocols.

3.2.2 Effects on Motor Cortical Inhibition and Facilitation

rTMS can also induce changes in cortical inhibition and facilitation. These changes can be assessed using single and paired pulse TMS paradigms including: (1) short-interval intracortical inhibition (SICI) (i.e., paired pulse TMS (ppTMS) at inhibitory interstimulus intervals (ISIs) of <5 ms) [19], (2) long-interval intracortical inhibition (LICI) [20, 21], and (3) silent period (SP) [22] methods (see Fig. 3.1). These inhibitory paradigms may measure different subtypes of inhibitory GABAergic neurotransmission [23]. Cortical facilitation can be measured using paired pulse TMS with interstimulus intervals between 10 and 20 ms, referred to as intracortical

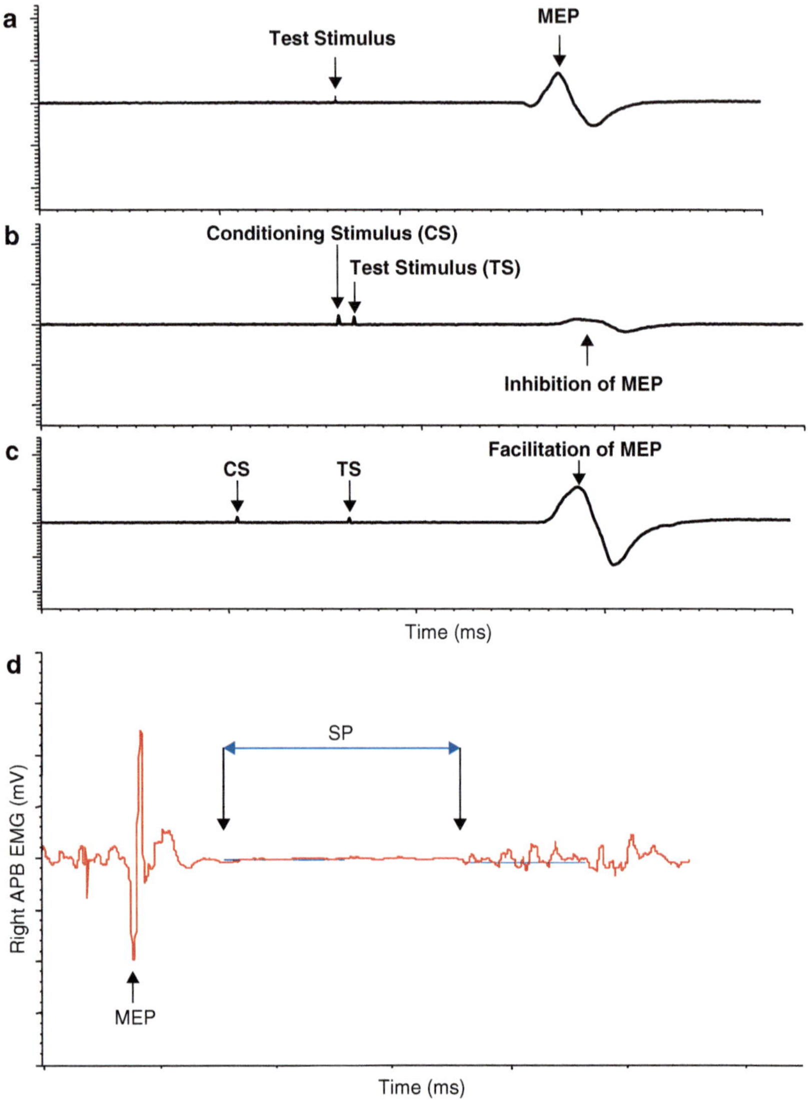

Fig. 3.1 Illustration of the assessment of the measures of short- and long-interval intracortical inhibition (SICI and LICI), cortical facilitation (CF), and the cortical silent period (SP). In the measurement of CF, SICI, and LICI, the motor evoked potential (MEP) response to a single test stimulus (**a**) is compared to the MEP response produced by a conditioning and test stimulus (**b** and **c**). When the conditioning stimulus is provided at a very short interval prior to the test stimulus (1–4 ms), the MEP produced a substantially reduced size (as illustrated in **b**) which is SICI. CF is produced when the interstimulus interval is between 10 and 15 ms and the MEP size is increased over the baseline measure (**c**). LICI is produced when the interstimulus interval is extended to 100 ms (not shown). The SP measure is demonstrated in **d**. The TMS pulse is applied when the corresponding muscle in the contralateral hand is undertaking a tonic muscle contraction. A period of suppression of tonic muscle activity is produced following the MEP and this is referred to as the silent period

facilitation (ICF) [19]. ICF may be mediated by glutamatergic neurotransmission [24].

Silent Period (SP)

The effects of rTMS on the SP have been investigated in several studies examining the effects of pulse number, stimulation frequency, and intensity. A silent period is mostly believed to assess activity of the $GABA_B$ receptor. Berardelli et al. [25] demonstrated lengthening of the SP with 3 and 5 Hz rTMS at 110% and 120% of the RMT. Romeo et al. [26] tested rTMS frequencies of 1, 2, 3, 5, 10, and 15 Hz at intensities just above the RMT. They found that trains delivered at ≥2 Hz resulted in a prolongation of the SP, whereas trains delivered at 1 Hz had no effect. In both studies, the authors suggested that the SP was prolonged because rTMS activated cortical inhibitory interneurons. Fierro et al. [27] explored the effects of 1 and 7 Hz rTMS at intensities of 100%, 115%, and 130% of the RMT. They found that 1 Hz rTMS applied to the motor cortex near or above the motor threshold reduced the SP. This was interpreted as a decrease in cortical inhibition. In contrast, 7 Hz rTMS resulted in an inconsistent pattern of smaller and larger values for the SP. The authors concluded that rTMS applied at low 1 Hz frequency decreases the excitability of inhibitory interneurons.

Therefore, it appears the effects of rTMS on the SP are dependent on frequency and intensity of stimulation. High-frequency rTMS (>1 Hz) results in lengthening of the SP, whereas low-frequency rTMS (~1 Hz) results in shortening of the SP. Moreover, at high frequencies, increasing the stimulus intensity results in further lengthening of the SP [28]. For example, for frequencies ranging from 1 Hz to priming (i.e., 6 Hz followed by 1 Hz), 10 and 20 Hz stimulation resulted in a prolongation of the SP. Twenty Hertz stimulation resulted in greatest prolongation of the SP. As the silent period was reported to be shortened in depression [29], this finding could help to identify the stimulation parameters needed to optimally treat depression. In fact, treatment with ECT in depression was associated with significant lengthening of the SP [30]. It is possible that both ECT and rTMS share similar mechanisms of action. For example, in Fig. 3.2 we illustrate how ECT induces seizures through direct activation of pyramidal neurons. Seizures terminate, in part, through activation of recurrent collaterals which activate GABAergic interneurons which could account for the SP prolongation seen with ECT. By contrast, rTMS activates interneurons transsynaptically [31], and this could result in a direct effect on GABAergic interneurons without causing a seizure.

Paired Pulse Inhibition and Facilitation (ppTMS)

The effects of rTMS on cortical inhibition and facilitation have also been evaluated through ppTMS. SICI assessed with ppTMS is widely believed to assess activity at the $GABA_A$ receptor. Pascual-Leone et al. [32] demonstrated SICI was significantly reduced with 1600 subthreshold rTMS stimuli applied at 10 Hz to the motor cortex. In contrast, the same number of subthreshold stimuli applied at 1 Hz had no effect on SICI. Similarly, Peinemann et al. [33] demonstrated that 5 Hz TMS applied to the motor cortex at 90% RMT caused a significant reduction in SICI but no change

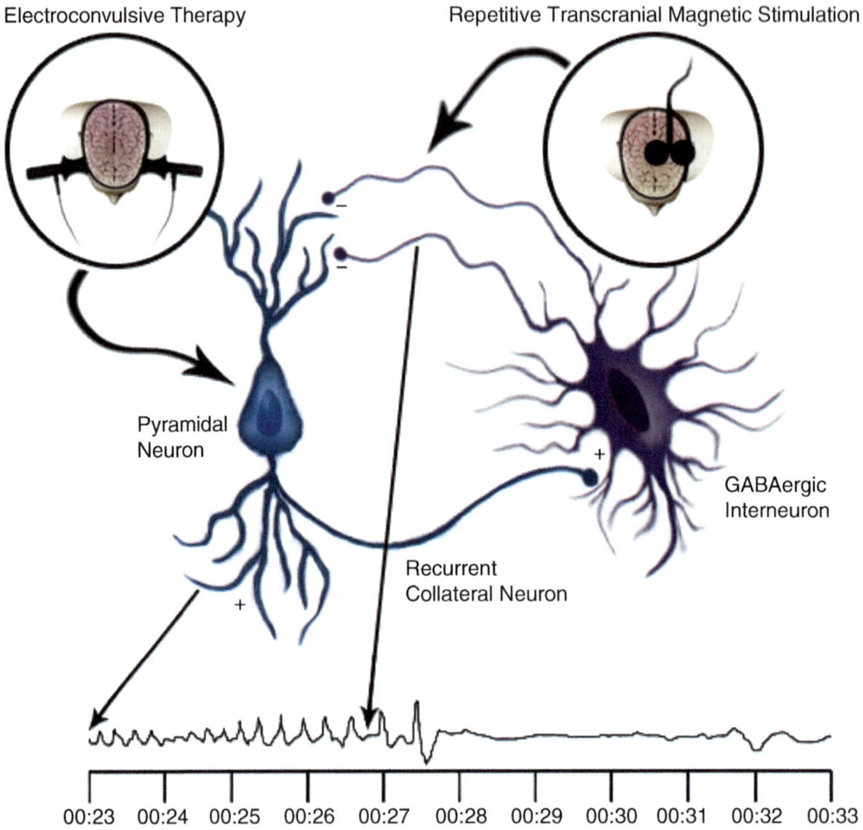

Fig. 3.2 Proposed mechanism for the role of GABAergic potentiation in the treatment of MDD. Cortical stimulation through treatments such as electroconvulsive therapy (ECT) results in rhythmic activation of pyramidal neurons with concurrent spike and wave complexes on electroencephalography (EEG). Subsequently, GABA interneurons are activated via feedback loops which attenuate cortical seizure activity, suppress EEG activity, and potentiate GABA inhibitory neurotransmission. Repetitive transcranial magnetic stimulation (rTMS) may exert therapeutic effects by transsynaptic facilitation of GABAergic neurotransmission in an analogous manner

in ICF. SICI was significantly reduced after only 30 stimuli of 120% RMT at 5 Hz [34]. Similarly, SICI was reduced at a stimulation frequency of 15 Hz, whereas ICF was increased. Romero et al. [6] found that subthreshold stimulation with 1 Hz for 10 min significantly decreased ICF, without a concomitant change in SICI. These authors suggest that these effects occur through cortical dysfacilitation. As ICF may be associated with activity of excitatory glutamatergic circuits [24], dysfacilitation may result in decreased cortical excitation. Therefore, these studies suggest that high-frequency rTMS decreases SICI and, perhaps, increases ICF. Conversely, low-frequency rTMS may decrease ICF without concomitant change in SICI.

The result of this series of studies exploring the effect of rTMS on SP and SICI suggests that rTMS modulates activity at both GABA receptor subtypes.

3.2.3 Effects of rTMS on Motor Cortical Plasticity

Repetitive TMS has also been shown to affect cortical plasticity. In this context, plasticity refers to the reorganization of the central nervous system (CNS) through changes in internal connections, representational patterns, and/or neuronal properties [35]. Ziemann et al. [35] demonstrated that the deafferented motor cortex becomes modifiable by inputs that are normally subthreshold for inducing plastic changes. Their findings suggest that rTMS can modulate plasticity and may potentially be used to enhance cortical plasticity when it is beneficial and suppress it when it is detrimental. In a subsequent study [36], lorazepam (which enhances GABAergic neurotransmission) and lamotrigine (which blocks voltage-gated Na^+ and Ca^{2+} channels) were found to abolish the increase in MEP size and decrease in SICI associated with concurrent ischemic nerve block and rTMS to the contralateral motor cortex. Conversely, dextromethorphan (NMDA receptor antagonist) suppressed the changes in SICI but had no effect on MEP. These results provide evidence that the increase in MEP size induced by rTMS and deafferentation both involve GABA-related inhibitory circuits and voltage-gated Na^+ or Ca^{2+} channel-mediated mechanisms. Also, rTMS-induced reduction in SICI appears to involve NMDA receptor activation.

The importance of these motor plasticity findings to the understanding of the mechanisms of rTMS in the treatment of depression is not fully clear. However, depression is a disorder associated with neural mechanisms putatively associated with plasticity impairments. For example, Levinson et al. [29] demonstrated that patients with depression had SP deficits, while patients with treatment-resistant depression had both SICI and SP deficits. These findings imply that depression is associated with deficits in GABAergic inhibitory neurotransmission, and that more treatment-resistant depression is associated with even more marked GABAergic inhibitory deficits. Further, several dimensions of depressive symptoms (e.g., memory deficits) may be associated with dysfunctional plasticity. Dysfunctional plasticity may also be a corollary to excessive NMDA receptor activation from chronic stress [37]. Additionally, deficits in brain-derived neurotrophic factor (BDNF) in depression may result in plasticity deficits, as BDNF serves to facilitate plasticity in the brain [38]. It may be possible that one of the mechanisms through which rTMS results in enhanced plasticity is the repetitive stimulation of neurons resulting in synchronous firing and long-term potentiation. That is, by repetitively stimulating neurons, neuronal output is strengthened and, over time, may translate into meaningful and more functional patterns of activity in depression.

3.3 Effects of rTMS Assessed with EEG

Assessment of immediate and direct rTMS-induced alterations in cortical activity can not only be assessed by electromyography (EMG) methods as described in previous chapters but also by electroencephalography (EEG). The use of the combination of TMS and EEG methods in the investigation of TMS mechanisms is particularly relevant for studies of working memory (WM) in depression. Abnormalities of WM have been repeatedly found in patients with MDD as well as a range of other psychiatric disorders. As discussed, rTMS over the motor cortex has been shown to enhance gamma (γ)-aminobutyric acid (GABA)-mediated inhibitory neurotransmission in healthy individuals [28]. Gamma oscillatory activity during higher cognitive tasks is an area of great interest and has recently been shown as a key neurophysiological mechanism underlying WM.

Commonly defined as the ability to maintain and manipulate information over short periods of time [39], WM is often argued as the essence of all prefrontal functions due to its importance in everyday complex cognitive tasks such as language, comprehension, learning, and reasoning [40, 41]. Moreover, the dorsolateral prefrontal cortex (DLPFC) is consistently reported to mediate WM processes, revealed through enhanced blood oxygen level-dependent (BOLD) activity in functional magnetic resonance imaging (fMRI) studies [42, 43]. It has been proposed that GABA inhibitory interneurons in the DLPFC contribute to the generation and synchronization of pyramidal neurons necessary for optimal WM performance [44, 45].

Investigating this issue, we previously conducted a study measuring the effect of 20 Hz rTMS applied to the DLPFC on γ oscillatory activity across WM load (i.e., 0-, 1-, and 2-back conditions) in healthy controls. Active rTMS significantly increased γ oscillatory activity compared to baseline (pre) and sham stimulation. Moreover, active rTMS caused the greatest change in γ oscillatory activity in the *n*-back conditions with the greatest cognitive demand, an effect that was limited to frontal brain regions. Finally, active rTMS had no effect on other frequency ranges (i.e., δ, θ, α, β), suggesting a selective effect to oscillatory activity in the γ frequency range. Collectively, these results suggest that active rTMS applied to DLPFC significantly increased frontal γ oscillatory activity which was most pronounced at *n*-back conditions of greatest difficulty. Therefore, it is possible that the effects of rTMS on DLPFC activity in depression may occur through modulation of high-frequency oscillations, and modulation of these oscillations may occur through alterations in the GABAergic neurotransmitter system.

3.4 Neuroimaging Studies of the Effect of rTMS

Part of the allure for studying the motor cortex is that outcome variables can be easily assessed with surface EMG. Exploring non-motor regions, however, requires combining TMS with other methods of measurement (e.g., EEG, positron emission tomography (PET), near-infrared spectroscopy (NIR), or magnetic resonance imaging (MRI)). A substantial series of studies have utilized brain imaging methods to either study the direct effects of rTMS stimulation (in a variety of cortical regions) or the effects of rTMS treatment in patients with depression.

3.4.1 Imaging of rTMS Effects

Studies directly imaging the effects of rTMS on brain regions have demonstrated that local activation of the cortex results in changes in distributed brain regions. For example, Paus et al. [46] stimulated the frontal eye fields with 10 Hz rTMS at an intensity of 70% of the maximum stimulator output while PET scans were acquired. They found significant positive correlation with regional cerebral blood flow (rCBF), as measured with ^{15}O-labeled H_2O PET over the same cortical regions, as well as concomitant excitation in the visual cortex of the superior parietal and medial parieto-occipital regions. In an alternative approach, Nahas et al. [47] used 1 Hz rTMS to stimulate the prefrontal cortex while functional MRI (fMRI) scans were conducted. This was done in an effort to measure connectivity and clarify the intensities that are required to produce activation in this cortical region. Previous studies measuring activation in non-motor cortical areas based intensities on those required to produce activation to the motor cortex [48]. Given the cytoarchitectural differences between these regions [49], however, such parameters may not be accurate. As such, the prefrontal cortex was stimulated with a range of intensities (e.g., 80%, 100%, and 120% of the RMT). Nahas et al.'s results can be summarized into four main findings: (1) greater intensities produced greater local and contralateral activation, (2) stimulation of the left prefrontal cortex resulted in bilateral effects, (3) rTMS of the left prefrontal cortex produced greater activation on the right side than the left side, and (4) stimulation at 80% of the RMT for 20 s failed to produce significant prefrontal activation.

An additional imaging approach used to study rTMS effects has utilized metabolic imaging with PET. With this method, Strafella et al. [50] demonstrated that rTMS applied to mid-dorsolateral prefrontal cortex resulted in dopamine release in the striatum of the human brain, indicating that rTMS applied to the cortex can induce neurochemical change in subcortical brain regions.

The most relevant conclusions from direct neuroimaging studies of rTMS to understanding the mechanism of action of rTMS treatment of depression are clearly that rTMS produces changes locally, and at distant brain sites within connected circuitry. This suggests the possibility that rTMS treatment may work through local effects, distal effects, or a combination of both. It is also quite plausible that the mechanism of action of rTMS may involve changing the strength of connections between areas in these brain circuits.

3.4.2 Imaging of rTMS Effects in Depression

Of more direct relevance to understanding the mechanism of action of rTMS treatment in depression are a series of studies that have examined brain activity pre- and post-rTMS treatment. Several existing lines of evidence suggest that MDD is more commonly associated with hypoexcitability over the left prefrontal cortex and/or hyperexcitability over the right prefrontal cortex. The strongest evidence in support of this relates to the much higher rates of depression in patients with left-sided strokes (the anatomic equivalent of hypoexcitability) than in the general population. Moreover, patients with right-sided strokes (the anatomic equivalent of hyperexcitability) experience manic symptoms at much higher rates than in the general population [51].

Imaging studies have also demonstrated that MDD may involve dysregulation of cortical activity, with lower activity in the left dorsolateral prefrontal cortex and higher activity in the right dorsolateral prefrontal cortex [52, 53]. Further, rTMS treatment in MDD has been directly shown to be associated with a normalization of hypoexcitability over the left prefrontal cortex and normalization of hyperexcitability over the right hemisphere [54]. This is consistent with the finding that rTMS applied at high frequencies (e.g., 10 Hz) increases excitability in the cortex [55], while rTMS applied at low frequencies (e.g., 1 Hz) decreases excitability in the cortex [3]. Specifically, Kimbrell et al. [54] reported that 13 patients with depression responded differently to 1 Hz versus 20 Hz rTMS. There was a significant negative correlation between change in HAMD scores and each frequency they were treated with. That is, responders to one frequency (i.e., 1 Hz or 20 Hz) tended to deteriorate when the other frequency was applied (i.e., 20 Hz or 1 Hz). Overall, however, there was a greater response to 1 Hz rTMS compared to 20 Hz rTMS. Additionally, in 11 patients who received PET scans, change in HAMD scores in response to rTMS was related to baseline glucose metabolism measures. Two weeks of 20 Hz rTMS was correlated with baseline global metabolism, with improved response associated with greater baseline global hypometabolism. Conversely, baseline global hypermetabolism was more closely associated with greater HAMD change scores following 1 Hz rTMS. The results suggest that brain metabolic biomarkers may be an effective way of optimizing or personalizing rTMS treatment response.

In addition to this initial PET research, studies have used a number of other methods to explore brain activity pre- and post-treatment. Research using functional magnetic resonance imaging (MRI) has indicated that high-frequency left-sided rTMS produces a bilateral prefrontal increase in task-related activation [56]. Interestingly, in the same study, successful response to low-frequency right-sided stimulation was associated with bilateral reductions in prefrontal activity. These bilateral changes suggest that successful response to rTMS treatment is not related to a simple rebalancing of left-right activity, and that response to treatment may involve alternative mechanisms. Interestingly in this context, recent studies have suggested that response to rTMS may be related to changes in white matter pathways in prefrontal-subcortical circuitry [57]. This research suggests that rTMS response does not necessarily relate to local changes in cortical activity, but arises through strengthening of cortical subcortical circuitry. Strengthening of these connections could potentially allow executive prefrontal cortical regions to exert greater regulatory control over abnormally active subcortical mood circuitry.

3.4.3 Studying Brain Effects of rTMS with Near-Infrared Spectroscopy

An alternative mechanism of exploring the effects of rTMS stimulation on brain activity is through the use of near-infrared spectroscopy (NIRS). NIRS is a technique for measuring blood oxygenation (HbO) that can be used in combination with rTMS and repeatedly over time. Initial research using NIRS to study the effects of single pulse TMS demonstrated quite consistently that higher intensity TMS results in a drop in HbO, both at primary motor cortex (M1) and at prefrontal cortex (PFC) (e.g., [58, 59]). Subthreshold single pulse TMS results in a more recognizable increase in HbO than would be expected to be seen during normal brain activation. More recent studies have found that the decrease in HbO that results from high-intensity TMS stimulation can also be seen with paired TMS pulses [59] and rTMS [60]. For example, we recently demonstrated that prolonged trains of 1 Hz rTMS at suprathreshold intensities produced a prolonged and sustained reduction in HbO not seen with subthreshold stimulation [61]. This pattern of substantial HbO reduction appears to be an "unnatural" pattern of brain activation, differing from what would be expected for normal brain activation or engagement in a cognitive task [58, 59, 61, 62]. Speculatively, it is possible that the brain's response to this unnatural pattern of brain activation, such as a change in vasomotor activity, may in some way underlie the therapeutic action of rTMS.

3.5 Studying Brain Effects of rTMS with Electroencephalography

EEG methods have been used relatively extensively to study aspects of rTMS treatment of depression. Initially EEG was used to investigate whether there were safety-related issues with rTMS treatment. More recently, a series of studies have investigated whether EEG markers can be used to predict successful response to rTMS treatment (e.g., [63, 64]). Of most relevance, however, are studies that have investigated changes in EEG activity associated with successful antidepressant treatment. For example, Spronk et al. evaluated the effects of rTMS applied over the DLFPC on quantitative EEG (QEEG) and the oddball ERP in patients with depression [65]. They reported that QEEG measures did not change with treatment, with the exception of an indirect right frontal increase in delta power. By contrast, rTMS resulted in an increased positivity in ERPs over the left frontal cortex. Specifically, the P2 amplitude was significantly increased in left frontal regions. There was also a treatment-related increase in N1 and N2 ERP components. These results suggest that rTMS can alter conventional neurophysiological markers of plasticity in the cortex. Such measures may ultimately serve as biomarkers of treatment response and help tailor or personalize rTMS treatment.

3.6 Effects of rTMS on BDNF

Given the postulated role of neurotrophic factors, including BDNF, in the etiology of depression and the mechanism of action of antidepressant medication, studies have increasingly explored whether the antidepressant effects of rTMS are modulated through rTMS-induced changes in BDNF. These studies have occurred both in animal models and in human experimental settings.

For example, high-frequency rTMS was shown to produce a substantial increase in BDNF levels in rats when stimulation was applied in awake animals, an effect not seen with low-frequency stimulation [66]. In a second study, 3 weeks of high-frequency stimulation was also shown to produce increases in BDNF levels along with changes in hippocampal cell proliferation [67]. In humans, Bocchio-Chiavetto et al. [68] reported that five daily sessions of rTMS administered to 16 patients with MDD resulted in significantly improved depression (average improvement by HAMD of 23.60%; $p = 0.0003$) with a concomitant increase in serum BDNF levels (baseline, 29.73 ± 8.02 ng/mL; post-treatment, 32.63 ± 7.59 ng/mL; $p = 0.022$). However, the clinical relevance of these findings is uncertain as the authors reported the increment in the neurotrophin levels was not associated with rTMS efficacy. Additional evidence from Lang et al. [69] also failed to detect an association of BDNF with clinical improvement following ten rTMS treatments of 14 patients suffering from treatment-resistant major depression.

The relationship of the BDNF system to rTMS response has also been explored in human subjects by considering the relationship between clinical response to treatment and BDNF genotype, specifically the effect of the val66met BDNF polymorphism. In a study of 36 patients where 31 had a diagnosis of major depression and the remainder 5 of bipolar disorder (depressive phase), 5 daily sessions of rTMS improved patient HAMD scores (baseline, 23.19 ± 5.12; post-rTMS, 17.50 ± 6.91; average = 25.29%). The val/val homozygotes (32.36 ± 21.23% improvement in HAMD) experienced a much greater improvement than met carriers (16.45 ± 19.90), indicating a role for this polymorphism in the improvement of depressive symptoms with rTMS treatment [68].

3.7 Conclusions

In summary, this chapter focused on rTMS mechanisms potentially associated with therapeutic improvement in depression. Treatment effects may relate to potentiation of excitatory and inhibitory cortical mechanisms. It is possible that rTMS responses relate to local changes in cortical activity, but also that response relates to an alteration of connections between prefrontal and subcortical brain regions relevant to depression. In addition, evidence suggests that rTMS may modulate plasticity in the cortex. Finally, both BDNF and dopaminergic increases have been reported, both of which have been related to the therapeutic mechanisms of rTMS. Future studies aiming to closely associate changes in these brain mechanisms to changes in symptomatic response may help clarify the physiological basis for the therapeutic effects of rTMS and potentially lead to optimized treatments.

References

1. Barker AT (1991) An introduction to the basic principles of magnetic nerve stimulation. J Clin Neurophysiol 8(1):26–37
2. Fitzgerald PB, Fountain S, Daskalakis ZJ (2006) A comprehensive review of the effects of rTMS on motor cortical excitability and inhibition. Clin Neurophysiol 117(12):2584–2596
3. Chen R, Classen J, Gerloff C, Celnik P, Wassermann EM, Hallett M et al (1997) Depression of motor cortex excitability by low-frequency transcranial magnetic stimulation. Neurology 48(5):1398–1403
4. Siebner HR, Auer C, Conrad B (1999) Abnormal increase in the corticomotor output to the affected hand during repetitive transcranial magnetic stimulation of the primary motor cortex in patients with writer's cramp. Neurosci Lett 262(2):133–136
5. Maeda F, Keenan JP, Tormos JM, Topka H, Pascual-Leone A (2000) Modulation of corticospinal excitability by repetitive transcranial magnetic stimulation. Clin Neurophysiol 111(5):800–805
6. Romero JR, Anschel D, Sparing R, Gangitano M, Pascual-Leone A (2002) Subthreshold low frequency repetitive transcranial magnetic stimulation selectively decreases facilitation in the motor cortex. Clin Neurophysiol 113(1):101–107
7. Muellbacher W, Ziemann U, Boroojerdi B, Hallett M (2000) Effects of low-frequency transcranial magnetic stimulation on motor excitability and basic motor behavior. Clin Neurophysiol 111(6):1002–1007
8. Fitzgerald PB, Brown T, Daskalakis ZJ, Chen R, Kulkarni J (2002) Intensity - dependent effects of 1 Hz rTMS on human corticospinal excitability. Clin Neurophysiol 113:1136–1141
9. Gerschlager W, Siebner HR, Rothwell JC (2001) Decreased corticospinal excitability after subthreshold 1 Hz rTMS over lateral premotor cortex. Neurology 57(3):449–455
10. Wassermann EM, Wedegaertner FR, Ziemann U, George MS, Chen R (1998) Crossed reduction of human motor cortex excitability by 1-Hz transcranial magnetic stimulation. Neurosci Lett 250(3):141–144
11. Chen R, Seitz RJ (2001) Changing cortical excitability with low-frequency magnetic stimulation. Neurology 57(3):379–380
12. Klein E, Kreinin I, Chistyakov A, Koren D, Mecz L, Marmur S et al (1999) Therapeutic efficacy of right prefrontal slow repetitive transcranial magnetic stimulation in major depression: a double-blind controlled study. Arch Gen Psychiatry 56(4):315–320
13. Pascual-Leone A, Valls-Sole J, Wassermann EM, Hallett M (1994) Responses to rapid-rate transcranial magnetic stimulation of the human motor cortex. Brain 117(Pt 4):847–858
14. Jahanshahi M, Ridding MC, Limousin P, Profice P, Fogel W, Dressler D et al (1997) Rapid rate transcranial magnetic stimulation—a safety study. Electroencephalogr Clin Neurophysiol 105(6):422–429
15. Berardelli A, Inghilleri M, Rothwell JC, Romeo S, Curra A, Gilio F et al (1998) Facilitation of muscle evoked responses after repetitive cortical stimulation in man. Exp Brain Res 122(1):79–84
16. Maeda F, Keenan JP, Pascual-Leone A (2000) Interhemispheric asymmetry of motor cortical excitability in major depression as measured by transcranial magnetic stimulation. Br J Psychiatry 177:169–173
17. Modugno N, Nakamura Y, MacKinnon CD, Filipovic SR, Bestmann S, Berardelli A et al (2001) Motor cortex excitability following short trains of repetitive magnetic stimuli. Exp Brain Res 140(4):453–459

18. Wang H, Wang X, Scheich H (1996) LTD and LTP induced by transcranial magnetic stimulation in auditory cortex. Neuroreport 7(2):521–525
19. Kujirai T, Caramia MD, Rothwell JC, Day BL, Thompson PD, Ferbert A et al (1993) Corticocortical inhibition in human motor cortex. J Physiol Lond 471:501–519
20. Valls-Sole J, Pascual-Leone A, Wassermann EM, Hallett M (1992) Human motor evoked responses to paired transcranial magnetic stimuli. Electroencephalogr Clin Neurophysiol 85(6):355–364
21. Wassermann EM, Samii A, Mercuri B, Ikoma K, Oddo D, Grill SE et al (1996) Responses to paired transcranial magnetic stimuli in resting, active, and recently activated muscles. Exp Brain Res 109(1):158–163
22. Cantello R, Gianelli M, Civardi C, Mutani R (1992) Magnetic brain stimulation: the silent period after the motor evoked potential. Neurology 42(10):1951–1959
23. Sanger TD, Garg RR, Chen R (2001) Interactions between two different inhibitory systems in the human motor cortex. J Physiol 530(Pt 2):307–317
24. Ziemann U, Chen R, Cohen LG, Hallett M (1998) Dextromethorphan decreases the excitability of the human motor cortex. Neurology 51(5):1320–1324
25. Berardelli A, Inghilleri M, Gilio F, Romeo S, Pedace F, Curra A et al (1999) Effects of repetitive cortical stimulation on the silent period evoked by magnetic stimulation. Exp Brain Res 125(1):82–86
26. Romeo S, Gilio F, Pedace F, Ozkaynak S, Inghilleri M, Manfredi M et al (2000) Changes in the cortical silent period after repetitive magnetic stimulation of cortical motor areas. Exp Brain Res 135(4):504–510
27. Fierro B, Piazza A, Brighina F, La Bua V, Buffa D, Oliveri M (2001) Modulation of intracortical inhibition induced by low- and high-frequency repetitive transcranial magnetic stimulation. Exp Brain Res 138(4):452–457
28. Daskalakis ZJ, Moller B, Christensen BK, Fitzgerald PB, Gunraj C, Chen R (2006) The effects of repetitive transcranial magnetic stimulation on cortical inhibition in healthy human subjects. Exp Brain Res 174(3):403–412
29. Levinson AJ, Fitzgerald PB, Favalli G, Blumberger DM, Daigle M, Daskalakis ZJ (2010) Evidence of cortical inhibitory deficits in major depressive disorder. Biol Psychiatry 67(5):458–464
30. Bajbouj M, Lang UE, Niehaus L, Hellen FE, Heuser I, Neu P (2006) Effects of right unilateral electroconvulsive therapy on motor cortical excitability in depressive patients. J Psychiatr Res 40(4):322–327
31. Rothwell JC (1997) Techniques and mechanisms of action of transcranial stimulation of the human motor cortex. J Neurosci Methods 74(2):113–122
32. Pascual-Leone A, Tormos JM, Keenan J, Tarazona F, Canete C, Catala MD (1998) Study and modulation of human cortical excitability with transcranial magnetic stimulation. J Clin Neurophysiol 15(4):333–343
33. Peinemann A, Lehner C, Mentschel C, Munchau A, Conrad B, Siebner HR (2000) Subthreshold 5-Hz repetitive transcranial magnetic stimulation of the human primary motor cortex reduces intracortical paired-pulse inhibition. Neurosci Lett 296(1):21–24
34. Wu T, Sommer M, Tergau F, Paulus W (2000) Lasting influence of repetitive transcranial magnetic stimulation on intracortical excitability in human subjects. Neurosci Lett 287(1):37–40
35. Ziemann U, Corwell B, Cohen LG (1998) Modulation of plasticity in human motor cortex after forearm ischemic nerve block. J Neurosci 18(3):1115–1123
36. Ziemann U, Hallett M, Cohen LG (1998) Mechanisms of deafferentation-induced plasticity in human motor cortex. J Neurosci 18(17):7000–7007
37. Pittenger C, Duman RS (2008) Stress, depression, and neuroplasticity: a convergence of mechanisms. Neuropsychopharmacology 33(1):88–109
38. Brunoni AR, Boggio PS, Fregni F (2008) Can the 'yin and yang' BDNF hypothesis be used to predict the effects of rTMS treatment in neuropsychiatry? Med Hypotheses 71(2):279–282
39. Baddeley A (1986) Working memory. Claredon Press, Oxford
40. Baddeley A (1992) Working memory. Science 255(5044):556–559

41. Baddeley A (2000) The episodic buffer: a new component of working memory? Trends Cogn Sci 4(11):417–423
42. Rasmussen KG, Knapp RG, Biggs MM, Smith GE, Rummans TA, Petrides G et al (2007) Data management and design issues in an unmasked randomized trial of electroconvulsive therapy for relapse prevention of severe depression: the consortium for research in electroconvulsive therapy trial. J ECT 23(4):244–250
43. Owens DS, Parker PY, Benton D (1997) Blood glucose and subjective energy following cognitive demand. Physiol Behav 62(3):471–478
44. Wang XJ, Buzsaki G (1996) Gamma oscillation by synaptic inhibition in a hippocampal interneuronal network model. J Neurosci 16(20):6402–6413
45. Traub RD, Michelson-Law H, Bibbig AE, Buhl EH, Whittington MA (2004) Gap junctions, fast oscillations and the initiation of seizures. Adv Exp Med Biol 548:110–122
46. Paus T, Jech R, Thompson CJ, Comeau R, Peters T, Evans AC (1997) Transcranial magnetic stimulation during positron emission tomography: a new method for studying connectivity of the human cerebral cortex. J Neurosci 17(9):3178–3184
47. Nahas Z, Lomarev M, Roberts DR, Shastri A, Lorberbaum JP, Teneback C et al (2001) Unilateral left prefrontal transcranial magnetic stimulation (TMS) produces intensity-dependent bilateral effects as measured by interleaved BOLD fMRI. Biol Psychiatry 50(9):712–720
48. Bohning DE, Shastri A, Nahas Z, Lorberbaum JP, Andersen SW, Dannels WR et al (1998) Echoplanar BOLD fMRI of brain activation induced by concurrent transcranial magnetic stimulation. Investig Radiol 33(6):336–340
49. Christensen BK, Bilder RM (2000) Dual cytoarchitectonic trends: an evolutionary model of frontal lobe functioning and its application to psychopathology. Can J Psychiatr 45(3):247–256
50. Strafella AP, Paus T, Barrett J, Dagher A (2001) Repetitive transcranial magnetic stimulation of the human prefrontal cortex induces dopamine release in the caudate nucleus. J Neurosci 21(15):RC157
51. Huffman JC, Stern TA (2003) Poststroke neuropsychiatric symptoms and pseudoseizures: a discussion. Prim Care Companion J Clin Psychiatry 5(2):85–88
52. Baxter LR Jr, Schwartz JM, Phelps ME, Mazziotta JC, Guze BH, Selin CE et al (1989) Reduction of prefrontal cortex glucose metabolism common to three types of depression. Arch Gen Psychiatry 46(3):243–250
53. Abou-Saleh MT, Al Suhaili AR, Karim L, Prais V, Hamdi E (1999) Single photon emission tomography with 99m Tc-HMPAO in Arab patients with depression. J Affect Disord 55(2–3):115–123
54. Kimbrell TA, Little JT, Dunn RT et al (1999) Frequency dependence of antidepressant response to left prefrontal repetitive transcranial magnetic stimulation (rTMS) as a function of baseline cerebral glucose metabolism. Biol Psychiatry 46:1603–1613
55. Pascual-Leone A, Valls-Sole J, Wasserman E, Hallett M (1994) Responses to rapid-rate transcranial magnetic stimulation of the human motor cortex. Brain 117:847–858
56. Fitzgerald PB, Sritharan A, Daskalakis ZJ, de Castella AR, Kulkarni J, Egan G (2007) A functional magnetic resonance imaging study of the effects of low frequency right prefrontal transcranial magnetic stimulation in depression. J Clin Psychopharmacol 27(5):488–492
57. Peng H, Zheng H, Li L, Liu J, Zhang Y, Shan B et al (2012) High-frequency rTMS treatment increases white matter FA in the left middle frontal gyrus in young patients with treatment-resistant depression. J Affect Disord 136(3):249–257
58. Thomson RH, Maller JJ, Daskalakis ZJ, Fitzgerald PB (2011) Blood oxygenation changes resulting from suprathreshold transcranial magnetic stimulation. Brain Stimul 4(3):165–168
59. Thomson RH, Daskalakis ZJ, Fitzgerald PB (2011) A near infra-red spectroscopy study of the effects of pre-frontal single and paired pulse transcranial magnetic stimulation. Clin Neurophysiol 122(2):378–382
60. Kozel FA, Johnson KA, Nahas Z, Nakonezny PA, Morgan PS, Anderson BS et al (2011) Fractional anisotropy changes after several weeks of daily left high-frequency repetitive transcranial magnetic stimulation of the prefrontal cortex to treat major depression. J ECT 27(1):5–10

61. Thomson RH, Rogasch NC, Maller JJ, Daskalakis ZJ, Fitzgerald PB (2012) Intensity dependent repetitive transcranial magnetic stimulation modulation of blood oxygenation. J Affect Disord 136(3):1243–1246
62. Mochizuki H, Ugawa Y, Terao Y, Sakai KL (2006) Cortical hemoglobin-concentration changes under the coil induced by single-pulse TMS in humans: a simultaneous recording with near-infrared spectroscopy. Exp Brain Res 169(3):302–310
63. Arns M, Drinkenburg WH, Fitzgerald PB, Kenemans JL (2012) Neurophysiological predictors of non-response to rTMS in depression. Brain Stimul 5(4):569–576
64. Narushima K, McCormick LM, Yamada T, Thatcher RW, Robinson RG (2010) Subgenual cingulate theta activity predicts treatment response of repetitive transcranial magnetic stimulation in participants with vascular depression. J Neuropsychiatry Clin Neurosci 22(1):75–84
65. Spronk D, Arns M, Bootsma A, van Ruth R, Fitzgerald PB (2008) Long-term effects of left frontal rTMS on EEG and ERPs in patients with depression. Clin EEG Neurosci 39(3):118–124
66. Gersner R, Kravetz E, Feil J, Pell G, Zangen A (2011) Long-term effects of repetitive transcranial magnetic stimulation on markers for neuroplasticity: differential outcomes in anesthetized and awake animals. J Neurosci 31(20):7521–7526
67. Feng SF, Shi TY, Fan Y, Wang WN, Chen YC, Tan QR (2012) Long-lasting effects of chronic rTMS to treat chronic rodent model of depression. Behav Brain Res 232(1):245–251
68. Bocchio-Chiavetto L, Miniussi C, Zanardini R, Gazzoli A, Bignotti S, Specchia C et al (2008) 5-HTTLPR and BDNF Val66Met polymorphisms and response to rTMS treatment in drug resistant depression. Neurosci Lett 437(2):130–134
69. Lang UE, Bajbouj M, Gallinat J, Hellweg R (2006) Brain-derived neurotrophic factor serum concentrations in depressive patients during vagus nerve stimulation and repetitive transcranial magnetic stimulation. Psychopharmacology 187(1):56–59

Acute rTMS Treatment for Depression

4

Abstract

A substantive series of clinical trials have supported the antidepressant efficacy of high-frequency rTMS applied to the left dorsolateral prefrontal cortex. The results of these trials have been summarized in several meta-analyses which support the positive antidepressant efficacy of this technique. Studies comparing rTMS and ECT have been substantially limited by sample size and design issues. In addition to high-frequency rTMS, studies have explored the use of low-frequency rTMS applied to the right dorsolateral prefrontal cortex and sequential bilateral rTMS combining both high- and low-frequency approaches with both showing efficacy in clinical trials and meta-analysis. Deep TMS, using a coil able to penetrate a significantly greater depth into the cortex, has also been shown to be effective as has stimulation with the novel theta-burst TMS paradigms. There are a number of significant methodological issues that need to be considered in evaluating rTMS trials and the application of this treatment. These include the method of coil localization and the way in which sham treatment is applied in clinical trials.

4.1 rTMS in Depression: High-Frequency Stimulation

When TMS was first used in the treatment of depression, single pulses were applied, often to the vertex, with minimal therapeutic benefit (e.g., [1]). However, it was not long before a more substantive and rational application of rTMS was developed. This application, which involved the stimulation of the left dorsolateral prefrontal cortex (DLPFC) with high-frequency rTMS pulses (Fig. 4.1), has persisted as the most common therapeutic paradigm until current times.

The rationale for high-frequency stimulation to the left DLPFC arose from the observation that patients with MDD exhibit a reduction in resting activity in the left

P. B. Fitzgerald, Z. J. Daskalakis, *rTMS Treatment for Depression*,
https://doi.org/10.1007/978-3-030-91519-3_4

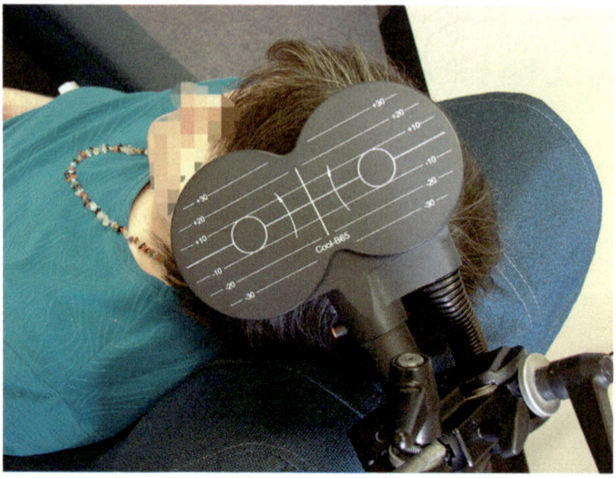

Fig. 4.1 A fluid cooled MagVenture A/S coil localized over the prefrontal cortex in the custom-built stand

DLPFC on positron emission tomography (PET) imaging [2]. A reduction in left prefrontal activity was also proposed to underlie the increased risk of depression following left anterior strokes, and there was also a suggestion of left-right anterior cerebral imbalance in electroencephalography studies. Early neurophysiological studies where rTMS was applied to the motor cortex had demonstrated that high-frequency stimulation would increase local cortical activity, usually assessed by the assessment of an increase, post-stimulation, in evoked motor activity to single TMS pulses. Therefore, it was proposed that high-frequency stimulation applied to the left DLPFC could increase local cortical activity and therefore ameliorate depression.

Initial studies using this technique in the mid-1990s produced considerable therapeutic benefit, despite the brief nature of the trials and relatively low dose of stimulation applied (e.g., [3, 4]). Subsequently, a very large number of open-label and single site sham-controlled trials have been conducted to explore the efficacy of left prefrontal rTMS (e.g., see Table 4.1). More than 30 trials have been sham-controlled although the methods for doing this have evolved over time. There has also been a progressive increase over time in the dose of rTMS stimulation applied during treatment and in clinical trials. This has manifested in changes in a number of stimulation parameters.

First, the intensity of stimulation has progressively increased. Initial trials typically applied stimulation at 90% or 100% of the resting motor threshold (RMT), whereas from the mid-2000s many trials used up to 120% of the RMT and this has become a de facto standard intensity in treatment application. The RMT is a measure of motor cortical excitability (see Fig. 4.2 and Chap. 12).

Second, the number of stimulation trains applied in each treatment session has also progressively increased. Initial studies provided 10 or 20 stimulation trains per session. Over time the number of trains progressively increased, and 75 trains per session have become the most commonly used approach following the pivotal trial that resulted in clinical approval of rTMS in the USA. Finally, the total number of stimulation sessions has also progressively increased. Treatment was initially

Table 4.1 Single site rTMS depression trials conducted between 1996 and 2006: a demonstration of the types of rTMS trials and representative results

Reference	Subjects	rTMS parameters	Significant difference: active vs. sham	Results
Avery et al. 2006 [57]	68 patients with treatment-resistant depression	15 sessions, delivered to the left dorsolateral PFC at 110% of the RMT (32 trains of 10 Hz repetitive TMS delivered in 5-s trains) Sham—45° coil tilt	Y	HRSD scores showed a significantly greater decrease over time in the TMS group compared with the sham group. Response rate for the TMS group was 30.6% greater than the 6.1% rate in the sham group
Berman et al. 2000 [58]	20 patients with treatment-resistant depression	10 sessions, 20 2-s trains of 20 Hz stimulation with 58-s intervals; delivered at 80% RMT Sham—45° coil tilt	Y	1 of 10 subjects receiving active treatment demonstrated a robust response (i.e., HRSD decreased from 47 to 7 points); 3 other patients demonstrated 40–45% decreases in HRSD scores. No patients receiving sham demonstrated partial or full responses
Cohen et al. 2003 [59]	10 patients with treatment-resistant depression	9 sessions over 2 weeks, 20 trains at 1.5 s at 20 Hz and 100% of the RMT over the left DLPFC followed by 2 trains of 60 s at 1 Hz and 100% of the RMT over the right DLPFC	n/a	4 of 10 subjects showed a ≥50% decline on the HRSD, with a strong trend for those under age 50
Conca et al. 2002 [39]	36 medicated depressed inpatients	Group 1: 110% of the RMT at 10 Hz over the left DLPFC, followed by 1 Hz stimulation of the right DLPFC at 110% of the RMT Group 2: stimulation of the left DLPC with alternating trains of 110% MT at 10 Hz and trains of 110% MT at 1 Hz in the same session Group 3: high-frequency stimulation over the left DLPC was performed as an internal control group	n/a	None of the treatment modalities was superior but different side effects were observed

(continued)

Table 4.1 (continued)

Reference	Subjects	rTMS parameters	Significant difference: active vs. sham	Results
Feinsod et al. 1998 [48]	10 patients with acute or residual schizophrenia	10 sessions, 120 stimuli daily at 1 Hz to right PFC, 9 cm round coil (100% RMT)	n/a	Significant decrease in BPRS score but in nonspecific items (anxiety, tension, restlessness)
Figiel et al. 1998 [48]	50 patients with refractory depression	5 sessions, 10 trains of 5 s with trains 30 s apart, 10 Hz stimulation at 110% of the RMT	n/a	21 responders (42%) based on final HRSD scores compared to baseline 56% of patients under age 65 responded and only 23% of those over age 65 responded
Fitzgerald et al. 2006 [41]	50 patients with treatment-resistant depression	3 trains of low-frequency rTMS to the right PFC of 140 s duration at 1 Hz were applied daily, followed immediately by 15 trains of 5 s duration of high-frequency left-sided rTMS at 10 Hz for 6 weeks Sham—45° coil tilt	Y	Significant decrease in MADRS scores for active treatment group at 2 weeks and across the full duration of the study. Those receiving active treatment met response (11 of 25 [44%]) or remission (9 of 25 [36%]) criteria by study end compared to the sham stimulation group (2 of 25 [8%] and none of 25, respectively)
Fitzgerald et al. 2003 [33]	60 patients with treatment-resistant depression	20 5-s HFL-TMS trains at 10 Hz and 5 60-s LFR-TMS trains at 1 Hz daily Sham—45° coil tilt	Y	Significant reduction in MADRS scores between the HFL-TMS and sham groups and between the LFR-TMS and sham groups
Geller et al. 1997 [60]	20 patients, 10 with schizophrenia and 10 with major depressive disorder	30 single pulses given in one session, 14 cm large round coil, bilateral PFC (100% RMT)	n/a	Several patients had short-lasting nonspecific improvement
George et al. 1997 [61]	12 depressed adults	20, 2-s, 20 Hz stimulations at 80% of the RMT over the left DLPFC Sham—45° coil tilt	Y	During the active phase, HRSD scores decreased significantly by 5.25 points

Table 4.1 (continued)

Reference	Subjects	rTMS parameters	Significant difference: active vs. sham	Results
George et al. 1995 [62]	6 medication-resistant depressed inpatients	Daily left PFC rTMS over several weeks	n/a	HRSD scores improved significantly for the group as a whole decreasing from 23.8 ± 4.2 (s.d.) at baseline to 17.5 ± 8.4 after treatment
Grunhaus et al. 2000 [21]	40 patients with major depressive disorder assigned to rTMS or ECT	rTMS: 20 sessions, 10 Hz for either 2 or 6 s for 20 trains at 90% of the RMT	n/a	Patients without psychosis responded similarly to both treatments and those with psychosis responded best to ECT
Hausmann et al. 2004 [40]	41 medication-free patients with major depressive disorder	10 sessions Group 1: active HFL-TMS of the DLPFC and subsequent sham LFR-TMS Group 2: simultaneous bilateral active stimulation (HFL-TMS and LFR-TMS) Group 3: bilateral sham stimulation (45° coil tilt)	N	No significant difference on the HRSD or BDI scores between groups There was a significant effect of time on all outcome variables in all groups (patients were administered an antidepressant on the first day of stimulation)
Klein et al. 1999 [31]	79 inpatients with major depressive disorder	10 sessions, 1 Hz, 0.1-ms pulse duration, at 10% above motor threshold (60 stimuli over 1 min) Sham—perpendicular coil tilt	Y	Significant reduction in depression scores as shown by the HRSD and MADRS after 2 weeks of active treatment
Loo et al. 2003 [38]	19 medication-resistant depressed patients	3 weeks, 15 Hz (5 s on, 25 s off) × 24 at 90% of the RMT Sham—coils on the head were inactive and a third coil out of the subject's view was discharged for acoustic effect	N	Significant difference in HRSD and MADRS scores for each group from baseline but no changes comparing active to sham treatment
Loo et al. 1999 [63]	18 medication-resistant depressed patients	4 weeks, 10 Hz, 110% of the RMT, 30 trains of 5 s each, 30 s apart Sham—45° coil tilt	Y	After 4 weeks of real treatment, significant linear trends indicated improvement in the scores on the HRSD, MADRS, and the BDI

(continued)

Table 4.1 (continued)

Reference	Subjects	rTMS parameters	Significant difference: active vs. sham	Results
Menkes et al. 1999 [64]	8 depressed patients and 6 controls	8 sessions over 6 weeks, right frontal SF-rTMS, 0.5 Hz at RMT	n/a	Significant antidepressant effect was noted in depressed patients on the HRSD and BDI scales. No change on either scale was noted in the controls
O'Reardon et al. 2007 [8]	301 medication-free patients with major depressive disorder	5 days/week for 4–6 weeks, 10 pulses per second at 120% of the RMT, 3000 pulses per session over the left DLPFC Sham—separate coil with embedded magnetic field	Y	Active TMS was significantly superior to sham on the MADRS at week 4 as well as HRSD at weeks 4 and 6
Padberg et al. 1999 [49]	18 patients with medication-resistant major depressive disorder	10 Hz, 0.3 Hz, or sham stimulation, 250 stimuli per day for 5 days at 90% of the RMT over the left DLPFC	N	Scores on the HRSD showed a significant time by group interaction; however, the effect was clinically marginal
Pascual-Leone et al. 1996 [4]	17 patients with medication-resistant depression	5 sessions, 20 trains of 10-s duration separated by 1 min pauses, 10 Hz at 90% of the RMT, positioned over vertex, left, or right DLPFC Sham—45° coil tilt	Y	Left DLPFC rTMS resulted in a significant decrease in scores on the HRSD and BDI

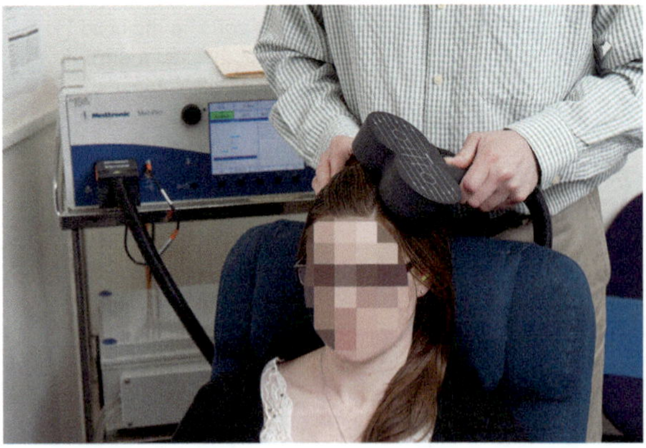

Fig. 4.2 Assessing the resting motor threshold using a handheld coil during stimulation of the motor cortex

provided over 1 or 2 weeks. This increased to 4 and then treatment trials of 6 weeks' duration were conducted, with some studies exceeding even this period [5].

Few studies have systematically addressed whether dose is directly related to clinical response. An inference has been made that the progressive increase in dose over time has been associated with an increase in efficacy reflected by greater effect sizes in later clinical trials [6]. However, it is possible that this increase has resulted from other factors, including changes in selection criteria for patients in clinical trials, and as these characteristics have increased simultaneously, it is not clear whether one or more of these dose-related factors is of greater importance. One recent large study compared dose—as defined by the number of rTMS pulses—for both high-frequency left-sided and low-frequency right-sided rTMS. One hundred and twenty-five trains of left-sided stimulation did not produce consistently better responses than 75 trains and no difference was seen between 20 min (1200 pulses) and 60 min (3600 pulses) of low-frequency right-sided rTMS [7]. Until further systematic research that randomizes patients to different dosage conditions is conducted, it is important to note that it remains an assumption that higher doses in most domains are associated with better clinical response although there seems the most consistent evidence that a greater number of treatment sessions are associated with better clinical outcomes. It is also worthy of note that the possible range of techniques that can be utilized in the application of rTMS have evolved considerably, for example, with the development of a variety of neuronavigational strategies for more accurately targeting prefrontal cortical regions. However, the vast majority of studies have generally used similar techniques to those developed in the mid-1990s. For example, the majority of studies establishing efficacy localized DLPFC by the measurement of 5 cm forward from the motor cortex in a sagittal plane. However, the methods used in clinical practice have somewhat diverged from this approach.

It is of some note that the vast majority of clinical trials conducted investigating the efficacy of rTMS have been independently funded and conducted by individual research groups. However, several larger-scale multisite sham-controlled trials have been published. The first of these studies was sponsored by an equipment manufacturer who had patent protection over a modified rTMS coil design (Neuronetics Ltd.). This study involved the randomization of over 300 medication-free patients to either active or sham stimulation [8]. Treatment was provided on a daily basis for 6 weeks which could be continued during a 3-week taper period. Seventy-five trains at 10 Hz were provided daily at a relatively high intensity. A non-identified sham stimulation coil system was used to ensure the blinding of both patients and clinicians. This trial demonstrated an antidepressant effect of active treatment compared to sham. However, this was not consistently found on all of the outcome measures, including the a priori nominated primary outcome measure. A substantial difference in antidepressant effect was seen depending on the degree of treatment resistance: patients who had not responded to only one antidepressant medication in the current episode responded to a substantially greater degree than those with a greater degree of treatment failure. Treatment was generally very well tolerated in this trial with no major adverse events. The results of this trial were used by the manufacturer to achieve device registration approval in the USA in 2008.

A second multisite US trial was funded independently by the National Institute of Mental Health and published in 2010 [9]. One hundred and ninety-nine patients were randomized to either active or sham stimulation which involved 3000 10 Hz pulses applied on a daily basis for 3 weeks, with a possible 3-week extension for partial responders. Similar methods were used to those applied in the Neuronetics Ltd.-sponsored study including the application of seventy-five 10 Hz trains at 120% of the RMT. Active stimulation produced a greater percentage of patients than sham stimulation who achieved remission of depressive symptoms although the overall rates of remission in both groups were low (14.1 vs. 5.1%). Treatment was also tolerated well in this study with a low dropout rate and no major adverse events.

We have been involved in the conduct of a series of large non-sham-controlled multisite trials investigating various rTMS stimulation parameters (e.g., [10, 11]). In these studies, when rTMS is applied in relatively heterogeneous but quite treatment-resistant samples of patients, we have generally found a response rate of approximately 50%.

4.1.1 Meta-Analysis

The results of a large number of studies exploring the efficacy of rTMS treatment in depression have been explored and summarized in a number of meta-analyses. The first meta-analyses of rTMS treatment in depression were actually published back in 2001 and 2002 although clearly, they included a relatively limited number of studies and subjects. Despite these small samples, the meta-analyses by McNamara et al. (5 trials) [12], by Holtzheimer et al. (12 trials) [13], and by Martin et al. (14 trials (n = 324)) [14] all found statistically significant evidence of antidepressant effects of rTMS treatment.

Significantly larger analyses were published later that decade and into the early 2010s. For example, the meta-analysis conducted by Schutter et al. [15] involved 30 trials and 1164 patients. The authors of this study found that there was a highly significant effect of active treatment compared to placebo, indicated by the average reduction in depression severity scores ($p < 0.00001$) with a moderate effect size (0.39). Interestingly, the degree of preexisting medication resistance and the intensity at which rTMS was applied did not affect outcomes. The authors of this study carefully evaluated the possibility of publication bias influencing analysis outcomes. There was no evidence of such a bias (non-publication of negative trials in the statistical analysis or the funnel plot). The authors concluded that approximately 270 unpublished negative studies would be required to counteract the positive results seen.

The meta-analysis conducted by Slotema et al. found similar results [16]. Thirty-four studies were analyzed comparing rTMS to sham stimulation (total n = 1383). The effect size was 0.55 ($p < 0.001$) and over 18,000 unpublished negative trials were found to be required for these results to have been produced by publication bias. Importantly, these authors found significant differences when rTMS was applied under different medication conditions. The overall effect size when rTMS was applied as a monotherapy was substantially higher (0.96, $p < 0.001$) than when rTMS was concurrently applied with medication (0.51, $p < 0.001$). The effect size was lowest when rTMS was started simultaneously with medication treatment (0.13, $p > 0.05$).

Over the last 10 years a considerable number of new meta-analyses have been published exploring the use of rTMS therapy but which have more focused on addressing specific questions about its application. For example, Teng et al. used meta-analytic techniques to demonstrate that greater antidepressant effects were achieved with longer periods of treatment but modest doses of stimulation per day [17]. Importantly, Wei showed that there was no difference between active and sham groups in regard to dropout rates in rTMS studies, indicating a high degree of acceptability and tolerability of treatment [18].

4.1.2 rTMS Versus ECT

In addition to trials exploring the efficacy of rTMS compared to sham stimulation, a number of trials have also compared high-frequency rTMS to ECT [19–24]. The majority of these studies report that rTMS has produced a similar degree of efficacy to ECT. However, these studies have not typically provided power analyses to indicate whether the studies have sufficient sample size to detect between-group differences and they are likely to be significantly underpowered to show differences between two active treatments.

The first of the rTMS/ECT comparison studies did demonstrate a difference between the treatments. In this trial, patients with psychotic depression showed greater benefit with ECT [22] although no differences were seen in patients without psychosis. A second more recent study also reported greater beneficial effects of ECT [25]. The overall results of these studies have been summarized using meta-analysis. This analysis included 6 studies ($n = 215$). It found that ECT produced a greater clinical benefit with an effect size of 0.47 ($p = 0.004$).

Despite these findings, it is important to note that the interpretation of studies comparing ECT to rTMS is very problematic. Almost all of these studies have compared a fixed number of unilateral rTMS treatments to a flexible course of often uni- and bilateral ECT. The number of rTMS treatments provided has often been relatively low compared to recent studies, and certainly rTMS has been rarely applied at what would not be regarded as a sufficient dose. In addition, no studies have allowed patients not responding to left-sided rTMS to cross over to right-sided or bilateral treatments, potentially the equivalent of converting from unilateral to bilateral ECT.

The question has also been raised as to whether comparing rTMS to ECT is really a substantially meaningful comparison [26]. We have argued that rTMS is more likely to be a complementary treatment provided to patients who do not require an urgent clinical response, which would suggest a need for immediate ECT, or in whom ECT is considered not suitable for safety or other clinical reasons. It is likely that rTMS will most frequently be offered to patients who are at early stages of treatment resistance or who have not quite the same degree of illness severity.

4.1.3 Network Meta-Analysis and Umbrella Reviews

Network meta-analysis is an approach to synthesizing data which involves the comparison of the outcomes that arise from multiple interventions in one single analysis. In this context, network meta-analysis has been used to compare the antidepressant benefits achieved with rTMS to other antidepressant strategies including antidepressant medication, medication augmentation, ketamine, and ECT. In an important study conducted by authors from the pharmaceutical industry, a variety of antidepressant strategies were evaluated for their effects at 2, 4, 6, and 8 weeks post-commencement of intervention [27]. In this analysis, rTMS was clearly the superior intervention at both 4 and 6 weeks (the times when rTMS outcomes are typically reported) when considering the overall results. Only rTMS and ECT were superior to placebo at 4 and 6 weeks and rTMS was ranked first in regard to actual rates of response and remission.

The antidepressant benefits of rTMS were also recently considered in an umbrella review, an approach that has been described as the highest form of evidence available for a treatment, which involves the synthesis of information from other systematic reviews and meta-analysis. This review [28], which used the rigorous GRADE approach to the assessment of the quality of evidence, concluded that there was "high-quality evidence" supporting the use of high-frequency left-sided TMS in the treatment of depression.

4.1.4 Real-World Data

In addition to data collected during clinical trials, valuable information on real-world effectiveness can be obtained from considering the results of treatment reported post-treatment implementation in standard clinical settings. A number of studies have reported these outcomes but the most impressive, published in 2020, reported on the outcomes of over 5000 patients from a substantial clinical register of outcome data. This outcome data was collected from patients treated in 103 practices and was reported based on an intention-to-treat (ITI) analysis as well as for treatment completers who received at least 20 rTMS sessions. Response and remission rates were quite impressive in both groups: 58% and 28% in the ITI group and 83% and 62% in the patients who completed at least 20 treatments. This supports the conclusion that substantive clinical outcomes are achieved with rTMS treatment in real-world clinical practice where patients are likely to diverge from those included in clinical trials in terms of their complexity and perhaps also in their capacity to follow through with rigorous clinical trial-based procedures, something of relevance given the intensive time-consuming nature of rTMS therapy.

4.1.5 Summary

A substantive series of single site and multisite research trials, supported by meta-analyses, have comprehensively established that rTMS applied at high frequency to the left DLPFC has antidepressant efficacy greater than sham and that these benefits are seemingly similar to, or better than, those seen with other treatments for patients who have failed initial antidepressant therapy, although we still lack a significant number of head-to-head trials comparing rTMS to other antidepressant strategies. One way to address this is to compare the effect sizes seen in trials to equivalent effect sizes seen with antidepressant medication strategies. O'Reardon et al. in their pivotal industry-sponsored clinical trial calculated that the number needed to treat (NNT) (number of patients needed to treat to get one responder) for rTMS was 12 at 4 weeks and 9 at 6 weeks [8], not dissimilar to the NNT for antidepressant medications [9] calculated from a large dataset [29]. It is worthy of note that a considerable number of rTMS trials have been conducted in patients with high rates of treatment resistance. Rates of remission with medication treatment in patients who have failed to respond to more than two antidepressants are very low, as demonstrated in the large STAR*D study, most likely substantially less than 20% (e.g., [30]).

4.2 Low-Frequency Right-Sided rTMS

High-frequency rTMS applied to the left DLPFC is not the only form of rTMS that has been systematically explored. Low-frequency stimulation (usually 1 Hz) applied to the right DLPFC has also been evaluated across a series of randomized controlled trials. In the first of these, conducted back in 1999, Klein et al. applied two relatively brief trains (1 min each), 3 min apart to the right DLPFC [31]. Patients were randomized to active or sham stimulation. Active stimulation was provided with a circular coil and generated a substantially greater improvement compared to sham stimulation. Since that time, a series of mostly relatively small studies have compared low-frequency right DLPFC stimulation to sham. These have used relatively divergent methods with some trials limited to 120 pulses applied by Klein et al., but others extending up to 1600 and 2000 pulses per treatment session. Most trials have utilized standard figure-of-eight shape coils.

The majority of these studies have shown positive antidepressant effects. This finding has been confirmed in a meta-analysis which demonstrated an effect size of 0.634 for active compared to sham stimulation [32] This result appears robust as approximately 120 negative studies would be required to render the effect significant. Notably, within this analysis, the authors compared the effect size apparent with low-frequency right-sided stimulation to that found in a previously conducted meta-analysis of high-frequency left-sided stimulation [15]. No differences were found, suggesting similar clinical effects. This is consistent with the findings of studies directly comparing the clinical effects of these forms of stimulation (e.g., [33]).

In fact, at least two meta-analyses have been published directly comparing the antidepressant benefits of high-frequency left-sided rTMS and low-frequency right-sided rTMS. Both of these have reported that there appears to be no significant difference in the overall clinical outcomes, whether assessing change in depressive symptoms, remission, or response rates [34, 35]. It is notable, however, that the vast majority of studies of low-frequency right-sided rTMS included in these analyses were done at lower doses of stimulation, in many cases at less than 120% of the RMT. However, we failed to find any differences between left- and right-sided rTMS in a large sample of 300 patients treated with high-dose/high-intensity protocols [7].

Of clinical relevance, response to one type of rTMS does not seem to exclude the possibility of response to the other [36]. It is also possible that there are differences in patients who would respond to either type, such that treatment could be individualized, but this has not been systematically investigated.

It is worthy of note that low-frequency stimulation should be safer than high-frequency stimulation as it reduces rather than increases cortical excitability, limiting further the risk of rTMS-related seizure induction [37]. As such, this might prove to be a useful therapeutic option in patients with increased risk of rTMS-related seizures. In our experience, across the conduct of the large number of clinical trials including both low- and high-frequency stimulation, generally low-frequency stimulation is better tolerated, associated with less scalp discomfort and fewer headaches. Occasionally patients who cannot continue with high-frequency stimulation have been able to receive a successful full course of low-frequency stimulation applied to the right DLPFC.

4.3 Bilateral rTMS

A third possibility that has been explored is the application of rTMS in a bilateral fashion. This has been driven both by the observation of the efficacy advantage of bilateral ECT and a motivation to take advantage of the efficacy of both right- and left-sided treatment approaches. The first study that explored bilateral rTMS applied simultaneous high-frequency stimulation to both sides of the brain [38]. No significant differences during 3 weeks of treatment were seen between active and sham stimulation in this study.

In contrast, the majority of subsequent bilateral trials have utilized the combination of low-frequency right-sided rTMS with high-frequency left-sided rTMS applied in a sequential fashion (sequential bilateral rTMS). The first study of this sort compared bilateral rTMS to high-frequency left-sided rTMS and a condition with high-frequency (10 Hz) and low-frequency (1 Hz) rTMS both applied to the left DLPFC [39]. No difference was found between the groups. However, this study was small, with a short 5-day period of treatment. A second study also showed no difference in response between bilateral and left-sided rTMS but rTMS commenced concurrently with antidepressant medication treatment [40]. In a study where sequential bilateral rTMS was directly compared to sham condition over a 6-week treatment period, a substantially greater response to active stimulation was seen compared to sham [41]. In this study, almost 50% of patients met response criteria and 36% met criteria for clinical remission.

Subsequent reports have continued to demonstrate the antidepressant benefits of sequential bilateral rTMS but not a consistent benefit of bilateral over unilateral treatment. One sham-controlled randomized study showed a greater response to bilateral compared to sham stimulation [42], but a similar sized study had exactly the opposite outcome [43]. In a much larger, but not sham-controlled, comparison, we found no difference between unilateral low-frequency right-sided rTMS and bilateral rTMS [10]. A second smaller study found an advantage of right over bilateral stimulation [44].

A number of meta-analyses have now been conducted exploring the effectiveness of bilateral TMS. In the first of these, bilateral rTMS was found to have greater antidepressant effects than sham stimulation and to have effects that appeared comparable to those of unilateral treatment [45]. Two network meta-analyses have been published that have investigated the relative benefits achieved with different forms of rTMS (either alone or considering other antidepressant strategies) [46, 47]. Both of these reported significant benefits of sequential bilateral rTMS, at least equivalent to other forms of rTMS therapy.

4.4 Other Approaches to Standard rTMS Treatment Delivery

There are potentially a variety of other approaches to the treatment of depression, some of which have been subject to limited evaluation. For example, although low-frequency stimulation has predominately been applied to the right DLPFC, several studies have suggested that low-frequency stimulation applied to the left DLPFC may have antidepressant effects [48–50]. We have also demonstrated that bilateral 1 Hz stimulation appears to have antidepressant activity [10]. One study has also investigated the effects of low-frequency stimulation applied to the right parietal cortex and suggested that this novel approach does have antidepressant effects [51].

Another approach that may have value is the use of a "priming" stimulation sequential combination. Priming stimulation involves the administration of a number of low-intensity high-frequency rTMS trains (usually subthreshold 6 Hz stimulation) prior to standard low-frequency rTMS [52] with this approach suggested on the basis of physiological experiments. The 6 Hz stimulation is proposed to "prime" the cortex and enhance the reduction in excitability produced by low-frequency stimulation. One study has shown that right-sided priming stimulation may be more effective than low-frequency right-sided stimulation applied alone [53] and its use was suggested to be potentially quite efficacious in one network meta-analysis {Brunoni 2017 #7089}. However, this approach has not been assessed in sham-controlled trials, and there may be other and potentially more effective methods of priming stimulation that have yet to be explored. For example, a recent approach has been developed using theta-burst stimulation (see discussion of this paradigm in the next section) to potentially prime the response to standard rTMS paradigms.

4.5 Issues with the Conduct of Clinical Trials of rTMS

One of the main issues with the conduct and interpretation of clinical rTMS trials from the outset has been the methodology of sham or placebo stimulation. All of the earlier rTMS trials used some variation of a method whereby a standard rTMS coil is placed on the head but angled away such that the majority of the produced magnetic field was not oriented toward the brain. If the coil is angled correctly, some degree of scalp nerve stimulation may be produced, mimicking in part the sensation produced with active TMS. The most common variations of this technique involved one of the two wings of the coil touching the scalp with the coil angled away from the scalp at either 45° or 90°. Studies investigating the capacity of this type of stimulation to act as an effective placebo were conducted in the early 2000s. For example, Lisanby et al. showed that tilting the coil away from the scalp from one wing would markedly attenuate the magnetic stimulation produced in the brain [54], and this method was widely adopted. They also demonstrated that tilting the coil forward across both wings did not substantially reduce the degree of intracortical stimulation; this approach should clearly be avoided.

In more recent years, a variety of new approaches have been developed and adopted. Neuronetics Ltd. developed an active and sham coil system for their pivotal registration trial, which involved the use of a known active coil for the measurement of motor thresholds followed by the randomization to either one of two coils, one of which was active and one of which was sham, for the provision of clinical trial treatment. The active and sham coils were identical in appearance in an attempt to maintain the blinding of treaters as well as patients. Another approach has been the development of combined TMS and electrical stimulation systems. In this approach, electrical stimulation of the scalp would be used to produce scalp sensation during sham TMS stimulation [55, 56]. Systems utilizing this approach are now commercially available, for example, from MagVenture A/S.

Variation in the quality of sham stimulation used in rTMS trials has led to some concern about interpretation of the results of many of these. Regardless of the form of sham stimulation utilized, the greatest reassurance about the quality of sham stimulation adopted can come when efforts are made to formally assess whether blinding has effectively been maintained. Studies are increasingly utilizing methods to assess whether patients have successfully remained blind although future research should also include adequate assessment of the blinding of raters and potentially treaters.

4.6 Conclusions

A variety of methods utilizing rTMS treatment for depression have been developed over the last 25 years. An extensive series of studies have evaluated the use of high-frequency stimulation applied to the left dorsolateral prefrontal cortex (see Table 4.2). This research clearly demonstrates the efficacy of this technique. There is also good evidence for the efficacy of low-frequency stimulation applied to the right DLPFC, although this form of rTMS has not been the subject of large-scale sham-controlled multisite trials, and sequential bilateral rTMS involving the use of low-frequency right-sided stimulation and high-frequency left-sided stimulation. The evidence suggests that these three approaches have relatively equivalent efficacy, and there is a preliminary data to suggest that patients may potentially benefit from a switch between approaches when failing to achieve an adequate response from initial treatment course. Several other approaches to the application of rTMS treatment including deep TMS and theta-burst stimulation will be explored in subsequent chapters.

Table 4.2 Evidence summary

Evidence type	High-frequency left	Low-frequency right	Sequential bilateral
Small single site sham-controlled trials	Yes	Yes	Yes
Multisite sham-controlled trials	Yes		
Meta-analysis	Yes	Yes	Yes
Network meta-analysis	Yes		
Umbrella review	High-quality evidence	Moderate quality evidence	High-quality evidence
Large real-world study data	Yes		

Summary of the evidence available for the three main forms of rTMS treatment

References

1. Grisaru N, Yaroslavsky U, Abarbanel JM, Lamberg T, Belmaker RH (1994) Transcranial magnetic stimulation in depression and schizophrenia. Eur Neuropsychopharmacol 4:287–288
2. George MS, Ketter TA, Post RM (1994) Prefrontal cortex dysfunction in clinical depression. Depression 2:59–72
3. George MS, Wassermann EM, Kimbrell TA, Little JT, Williams WE, Danielson AL et al (1997) Mood improvement following daily left prefrontal repetitive transcranial magnetic stimulation in patients with depression: a placebo-controlled crossover trial. Am J Psychiatry 154(12):1752–1756
4. Pascual-Leone A, Rubio B, Pallardo F, Catala MD (1996) Rapid-rate transcranial magnetic stimulation of the left dorsolateral prefrontal cortex in drug-resistant depression. Lancet 348:233–237
5. Daskalakis ZJ, Levinson AJ, Fitzgerald PB (2008) Repetitive transcranial magnetic stimulation for major depressive disorder: a review. Can J Psychiatr 53(9):555–566
6. Gross M, Nakamura L, Pascual-Leone A, Fregni F (2007) Has repetitive transcranial magnetic stimulation (rTMS) treatment for depression improved? A systematic review and meta-analysis comparing the recent vs. the earlier rTMS studies. Acta Psychiatr Scand 116(3):165–173
7. Fitzgerald PB, Hoy KE, Reynolds J, Singh A, Gunewardene R, Slack C, et al (2020) A pragmatic randomized controlled trial exploring the relationship between pulse number and response to repetitive transcranial magnetic stimulation treatment in depression. Brain Stimul 13(1):145–152
8. O'Reardon JP, Solvason HB, Janicak PG, Sampson S, Isenberg KE, Nahas Z et al (2007) Efficacy and safety of transcranial magnetic stimulation in the acute treatment of major depression: a multisite randomized controlled trial. Biol Psychiatry 62(11):1208–1216
9. George MS, Lisanby SH, Avery D, McDonald WM, Durkalski V, Pavlicova M et al (2010) Daily left prefrontal transcranial magnetic stimulation therapy for major depressive disorder: a sham-controlled randomized trial. Arch Gen Psychiatry 67(5):507–516
10. Fitzgerald PB, Hoy K, Gunewardene R, Slack C, Ibrahim S, Bailey M et al (2010) A randomized trial of unilateral and bilateral prefrontal cortex transcranial magnetic stimulation in treatment-resistant major depression. Psychol Med 7:1–10
11. Fitzgerald PB, Huntsman S, Gunewardene R, Kulkarni J, Daskalakis ZJ (2006) A randomized trial of low-frequency right-prefrontal-cortex transcranial magnetic stimulation as augmentation in treatment-resistant major depression. Int J Neuropsychopharmacol 9(6):655–666
12. McNamara B, Ray JL, Arthurs J, Boniface S (2001) Transcranial magnetic stimulation for depression and other psychiatric disorders. Psychol Med 31(7):1141–6
13. Holtzheimer PE, 3rd, Russo J, Avery DH (2001) A meta-analysis of repetitive transcranial magnetic stimulation in the treatment of depression. Psychopharmacol Bull 35(4):149–69
14. Martin JL, Barbanoj MJ, Schlaepfer TE, Clos S, Perez V, Kulisevsky J, et al (2002) Transcranial magnetic stimulation for treating depression. Cochrane Database Syst Rev (2):CD003493
15. Schutter DJ (2009) Antidepressant efficacy of high-frequency transcranial magnetic stimulation over the left dorsolateral prefrontal cortex in double-blind sham-controlled designs: a meta-analysis. Psychol Med 39(1):65–75
16. Slotema CW, Blom JD, Hoek HW, Sommer IE (2010) Should we expand the toolbox of psychiatric treatment methods to include Repetitive Transcranial Magnetic Stimulation (rTMS)? A meta-analysis of the efficacy of rTMS in psychiatric disorders. J Clin Psychiatry 71(7):873–884
17. Teng S, Guo Z, Peng H, Xing G, Chen H, He B, et al (2017) High-frequency repetitive transcranial magnetic stimulation over the left DLPFC for major depression: Session-dependent efficacy: A meta-analysis. Eur Psychiatry 41:75–84
18. Wei Y, Zhu J, Pan S, Su H, Li H, Wang J (2017) Meta-analysis of the Efficacy and Safety of Repetitive Transcranial Magnetic Stimulation (rTMS) in the Treatment of Depression. Shanghai Arch Psychiatry 29(6):328–342

19. Pridmore S, Bruno R, Turnier-Shea Y, Reid P, Rybak M (2000) Comparison of unlimited numbers of rapid transcranial magnetic stimulation (rTMS) and ECT treatment sessions in major depressive episode. Int J Neuropsychopharmacol 3(2):129–134
20. Janicak PG, Dowd SM, Martis B, Alam D, Beedle D, Krasuski J et al (2002) Repetitive transcranial magnetic stimulation versus electroconvulsive therapy for major depression: preliminary results of a randomized trial. Biol Psychiatry 51(8):659–667
21. Grunhaus L, Dannon PN, Schreiber S, Dolberg OH, Amiaz R, Ziv R et al (2000) Repetitive transcranial magnetic stimulation is as effective as electroconvulsive therapy in the treatment of nondelusional major depressive disorder: an open study. Biol Psychiatry 47(4):314–324
22. Grunhaus L, Dannon P, Schreiber S (1998) Effects of transcranial magnetic stimulation on severe depression. Similarities with ECT. Biol Psychiatry 43:76S
23. Eranti S, Mogg A, Pluck G, Landau S, Purvis R, Brown RG et al (2007) A randomized, controlled trial with 6-month follow-up of repetitive transcranial magnetic stimulation and electroconvulsive therapy for severe depression. Am J Psychiatry 164(1):73–81
24. Rosa MA, Gattaz WF, Pascual-Leone A, Fregni F, Rosa MO, Rumi DO et al (2006) Comparison of repetitive transcranial magnetic stimulation and electroconvulsive therapy in unipolar non-psychotic refractory depression: a randomized, single-blind study. Int J Neuropsychopharmacol 9(6):667–676
25. McLoughlin DM, Mogg A, Eranti S, Pluck G, Purvis R, Edwards D et al (2007) The clinical effectiveness and cost of repetitive transcranial magnetic stimulation versus electroconvulsive therapy in severe depression: a multicentre pragmatic randomised controlled trial and economic analysis. Health Technol Assess 11(24):1–54
26. Fitzgerald P (2004) Repetitive transcranial magnetic stimulation and electroconvulsive therapy: complementary or competitive therapeutic options in depression? Australas Psychiatry 12(3):234–238
27. Papadimitropoulou K, Vossen C, Karabis A, Donatti C, Kubitz N (2017) Comparative efficacy and tolerability of pharmacological and somatic interventions in adult patients with treatment-resistant depression: a systematic review and network meta-analysis. Curr Med Res Opin 33(4):701–711
28. Razza LB, Afonso Dos Santos L, Borrione L, Bellini H, Branco LC, Cretaz E, et al (2020) Appraising the effectiveness of electrical and magnetic brain stimulation techniques in acute major depressive episodes: an umbrella review of meta-analyses of randomized controlled trials. Braz J Psychiatry
29. Thase ME, Haight BR, Richard N, Rockett CB, Mitton M, Modell JG et al (2005) Remission rates following antidepressant therapy with bupropion or selective serotonin reuptake inhibitors: a meta-analysis of original data from 7 randomized controlled trials. J Clin Psychiatry 66(8):974–981
30. Fava M, Rush AJ, Wisniewski SR, Nierenberg AA, Alpert JE, McGrath PJ et al (2006) A comparison of mirtazapine and nortriptyline following two consecutive failed medication treatments for depressed outpatients: a STAR*D report. Am J Psychiatry 163(7):1161–1172
31. Klein E, Kolsky Y, Puyerovsky M, Koren D, Chistyakov A, Feinsod M (1999) Right prefrontal slow repetitive transcranial magnetic stimulation in schizophrenia: a double-blind sham-controlled pilot study. Biol Psychiatry 46(10):1451–1454
32. Schutter DJ (2010) Quantitative review of the efficacy of slow-frequency magnetic brain stimulation in major depressive disorder. Psychol Med 40(11):1789–1795
33. Fitzgerald PB, Brown T, Marston NAU, Daskalakis ZJ, Kulkarni J (2003) A double-blind placebo controlled trial of transcranial magnetic stimulation in the treatment of depression. Arch Gen Psychiatry 60:1002–1008
34. Cao X, Deng C, Su X, Guo Y (2018) Response and Remission Rates Following High-Frequency vs. Low-Frequency Repetitive Transcranial Magnetic Stimulation (rTMS) Over Right DLPFC for Treating Major Depressive Disorder (MDD): A Meta-Analysis of Randomized, Double-Blind Trials. Front Psychiatry 9:413

35. Chen J, Zhou C, Wu B, Wang Y, Li Q, Wei Y, et al (2013) Left versus right repetitive transcranial magnetic stimulation in treating major depression: a meta-analysis of randomised controlled trials. Psychiatry Res 210(3):1260–4.
36. Fitzgerald PB, McQueen S, Herring S, Hoy K, Segrave R, Kulkarni J et al (2009) A study of the effectiveness of high-frequency left prefrontal cortex transcranial magnetic stimulation in major depression in patients who have not responded to right-sided stimulation. Psychiatry Res 169(1):12–15
37. Fitzgerald PB, Fountain S, Daskalakis ZJ (2006) A comprehensive review of the effects of rTMS on motor cortical excitability and inhibition. Clin Neurophysiol 117(12):2584–2596
38. Loo CK, Mitchell PB, Croker VM, Malhi GS, Wen W, Gandevia SC et al (2003) Double-blind controlled investigation of bilateral prefrontal transcranial magnetic stimulation for the treatment of resistant major depression. Psychol Med 33(1):33–40
39. Conca A, Di Pauli J, Beraus W, Hausmann A, Peschina W, Schneider H et al (2002) Combining high and low frequencies in rTMS antidepressive treatment: preliminary results. Hum Psychopharmacol 17(7):353–356
40. Hausmann A, Kemmler G, Walpoth M, Mechtcheriakov S, Kramer-Reinstadler K, Lechner T et al (2004) No benefit derived from repetitive transcranial magnetic stimulation in depression: a prospective, single centre, randomised, double blind, sham controlled "add on" trial. J Neurol Neurosurg Psychiatry 75(2):320–322
41. Fitzgerald PB, Benitez J, de Castella A, Daskalakis ZJ, Brown TL, Kulkarni J (2006) A randomized, controlled trial of sequential bilateral repetitive transcranial magnetic stimulation for treatment-resistant depression. Am J Psychiatry 163(1):88–94
42. Blumberger DM, Mulsant BH, Fitzgerald PB, Rajji TK, Ravindran AV, Young LT et al (2012) A randomized double-blind sham-controlled comparison of unilateral and bilateral repetitive transcranial magnetic stimulation for treatment-resistant major depression. World J Biol Psychiatry 13(6):423–435
43. Fitzgerald PB, Hoy KE, Herring SE, McQueen S, Peachey AV, Segrave RA et al (2012) A double blind randomized trial of unilateral left and bilateral prefrontal cortex transcranial magnetic stimulation in treatment resistant major depression. J Affect Disord 139(2):193–198
44. Pallanti S, Bernardi S, Di Rollo A, Antonini S, Quercioli L (2010) Unilateral low frequency versus sequential bilateral repetitive transcranial magnetic stimulation: is simpler better for treatment of resistant depression? Neuroscience 167(2):323–328
45. Berlim MT, Van den Eynde F, Daskalakis ZJ (2013) A systematic review and meta-analysis on the efficacy and acceptability of bilateral repetitive transcranial magnetic stimulation (rTMS) for treating major depression. Psychol Med 43(11):2245–54
46. Brunoni AR, Chaimani A, Moffa AH, Razza LB, Gattaz WF, Daskalakis ZJ, et al (2017) Repetitive Transcranial Magnetic Stimulation for the Acute Treatment of Major Depressive Episodes: A Systematic Review With Network Meta-analysis. JAMA Psychiatry 74(2):143–152
47. Li H, Cui L, Li J, Liu Y, Chen Y (2021) Comparative efficacy and acceptability of neuromodulation procedures in the treatment of treatment-resistant depression: a network meta-analysis of randomized controlled trials. J Affect Disord 287:115–124
48. Figiel GS, Epstein C, McDonald WM, Amazon-Leece J, Figiel L, Saldivia A, et al (1998) The use of rapid-rate transcranial magnetic stimulation (rTMS) in refractory depressed patients. J Neuropsychiatry Clin Neurosci 10(1):20–5
49. Padberg F, Zwanzger P, Thoma H, Kathmann N, Haag C, Greenberg BD et al (1999) Repetitive transcranial magnetic stimulation (rTMS) in pharmacotherapy-refractory major depression: comparative study of fast, slow and sham rTMS. Psychiatry Res 88(3):163–171
50. Speer AM, Benson BE, Kimbrell TK, Wassermann EM, Willis MW, Herscovitch P et al (2009) Opposite effects of high and low frequency rTMS on mood in depressed patients: relationship to baseline cerebral activity on PET. J Affect Disord 115(3):386–394
51. Schutter DJ, Laman DM, van Honk J, Vergouwen AC, Koerselman GF (2009) Partial clinical response to 2 weeks of 2 Hz repetitive transcranial magnetic stimulation to the right parietal cortex in depression. Int J Neuropsychopharmacol 12(5):643–650

52. Iyer MB, Schleper N, Wassermann EM (2003) Priming stimulation enhances the depressant effect of low-frequency repetitive transcranial magnetic stimulation. J Neurosci 23(34):10867–10872
53. Fitzgerald PB, Hoy K, McQueen S, Herring S, Segrave R, Been G et al (2008) Priming stimulation enhances the effectiveness of low-frequency right prefrontal cortex transcranial magnetic stimulation in major depression. J Clin Psychopharmacol 28(1):52–58
54. Lisanby SH, Gutman D, Luber B, Schroeder C, Sackeim HA (2001) Sham TMS: intracerebral measurement of the induced electrical field and the induction of motor-evoked potentials. Biol Psychiatry 49(5):460–463
55. Borckardt JJ, Walker J, Branham RK, Rydin-Gray S, Hunter C, Beeson H et al (2008) Development and evaluation of a portable sham TMS system. Brain Stimulat 1(1):52–59
56. Mennemeier M, Triggs W, Chelette K, Woods A, Kimbrell T, Dornhoffer J (2009) Sham transcranial magnetic stimulation using electrical stimulation of the scalp. Brain Stimulat 2(3):168–173
57. Avery DH, Holtzheimer PE III, Fawaz W, Russo J, Neumaier J, Dunner DL et al (2006) A controlled study of repetitive transcranial magnetic stimulation in medication-resistant major depression. Biol Psychiatry 59(2):187–194
58. Berman RM, Narasimhan M, Sanacora G, Miano AP, Hoffman RE, Hu XS et al (2000) A randomized clinical trial of repetitive transcranial magnetic stimulation in the treatment of major depression. Biol Psychiatry 47(4):332–337
59. Cohen CI, Amassian VE, Akande B, Maccabee PJ (2003) The efficacy and safety of bilateral rTMS in medication-resistant depression. J Clin Psychiatry 64(5):613–614
60. Geller V, Grisaru N, Abarbanel JM, Lemberg T, Belmaker RH (1997) Slow magnetic stimulation of prefrontal cortex in depression and schizophrenia. Prog Neuropsychopharmacol Biol Psychiatry 21(1):105–110
61. George MS, Wasserman EM, Kimbrell TA et al (1997) Mood improvement following daily left prefrontal repetitive transcranial magnetic stimulation in patients with depression: a placebo-controlled crossover trial. Am J Psychiatry 154:1752–1756
62. George MS, Wassermann EM, Williams WA, Callahan A, Ketter TA, Basser P et al (1995) Daily repetitive transcranial magnetic stimulation (rTMS) improves mood in depression. Neuroreport 6:1853–1856
63. Loo C, Mitchell P, Sachdev P, McDarmont B, Parker G, Gandevia S (1999) Double-blind controlled investigation of transcranial magnetic stimulation for the treatment of resistant major depression. Am J Psychiatry 156:946–948
64. Menkes DL, Bodnar P, Ballesteros RA, Swenson MR (1999) Right frontal lobe slow frequency repetitive transcranial magnetic stimulation (SF r-TMS) is an effective treatment for depression: a case-control pilot study of safety and efficacy. J Neurol Neurosurg Psychiatry 67:113–115

5 Clinical Indications and Patient Selection

Abstract

A variety of issues need to be considered and comprehensively assessed when evaluating a patient for rTMS treatment. There is evidence in the literature suggesting that a number of individual illness characteristics are related to clinical response, including the degree of patient treatment resistance and age. Although there is evidence that treatment response is greater for patients with a lesser degree of treatment resistance and younger age, studies have shown antidepressant effects in patients who are considerably treatment resistant and of old age, and these factors do not appear to be sufficiently reliable to predict response, or nonresponse, to treatment. Although few studies have explicitly explored the use of rTMS in bipolar depression, studies have included bipolar depressed patients in mixed samples with no indication that bipolarity is associated with poor treatment response. There is limited evidence for the efficacy of rTMS in adolescents. Special consideration needs to be given when considering the use of rTMS treatment in special populations including pregnant women, women who are breastfeeding, or individuals affected by comorbid neurological disorders.

5.1 Stage of Illness and Treatment Resistance

There are a variety of times during the evolution of depressive illness when patients may potentially present for rTMS treatment. This could include during an initial episode of depression, during depressive relapse, during a period of persistent treatment-resistant depression, or possibly well when presenting for maintenance therapy. There is varying depth in the data that informs the use of rTMS across differing illness stages. It is reasonable to extrapolate potential efficacy across these stages, but sensible decisions about the likelihood of response should be based upon

P. B. Fitzgerald, Z. J. Daskalakis, *rTMS Treatment for Depression*, https://doi.org/10.1007/978-3-030-91519-3_5

the balanced judgment of the accumulated experience of rTMS treatment in the stage of illness being considered.

There are a variety of established treatment options for patients with depressive disorders. Approximately 40% of patients with an index episode of depression will respond to a single course of an antidepressant treatment and an additional estimated 30% to multiple antidepressants and augmentation strategies [1]. Systematic, equivalent data on response rates to psychological treatments is not available. However, it is reasonable to assume that a substantial proportion of individuals will not be suitable for these approaches or will continue to experience depressive symptoms despite adequate therapy. These groups of patients are typically regarded as having treatment-resistant depression (TRD). It is worthy of note that treatment outcomes for patients with TRD with standard treatment options are quite poor. For example, in an analysis of the STAR-D data, Sackeim showed that the likelihood of persistent benefit over 12 months being achieved via antidepressant medication once a patient has failed two initial medication trials is less than 5% [2].

Patients with treatment-resistant depression have been the focus of substantial bulk of the rTMS antidepressant research. However, there is considerable variation in methods used to define TRD [3], and this has affected the consistency and clarity of the definition of patient populations across treatment trials. Some trials have considered treatment-resistant patients as those who have failed as few as one or two antidepressant medication trials. Stricter definitions expand the number of failed trials and/or require these to have come from at least two separate medication classes. Tools such as the Antidepressant Treatment History Form (ATHF), the Thase and Rush Staging Model (TRSM), and the Massachusetts General Hospital Staging model (MGH-S) have been developed to assist in the characterization of individuals as treatment resistant, but have differing psychometric properties [4]. However, any of these are likely to be helpful in the process of the assessment of patients for rTMS treatment. It is important to gain information on a series of clinical features of past treatment failure as part of this process (see Box 5.1).

Box 5.1 Characteristics of Previous Biological Treatment Trials

1. Number of medication trials in current episode
2. Number of lifetime failed trials
3. Duration of each trial
4. Degree of clinical response (absent/partial/complete)
5. Maximal dose of medication prescribed in relation to therapeutic and maximally recommended doses
6. Number of drug classes covered by medication trials
7. Number of augmentation strategies
8. Characteristics of ECT courses: laterality, stimulation location, pulse parameters, number of treatments, seizure accuracy

Despite a large number of early rTMS trials having been conducted in patients who have failed a substantial number of medication trials, initial registration for rTMS in the USA was based on data from a comparison of antidepressant response between rTMS and sham stimulation in patients who had failed to respond to only one antidepressant medication. The approved indication for the use of rTMS expanded later to include a greater range of treatment resistance, but it is likely that this process created an impression for many that rTMS was predominately effective in those patients with a very limited degree of treatment resistance. There is certainly some evidence in the literature that a lesser number of failed medication trials is a positive predictor of likely antidepressant response (e.g., [5, 6]). However, several large studies have failed to confirm this relationship (e.g., [7]). On the basis of this literature, although it would seem to be favorable to make rTMS treatment available relatively early in the course of a treatment history—patients who are less treatment resistant are probably numerically more likely to respond—there is little evidence to suggest that patients should be excluded or dissuaded from treatment when they have failed a greater number of treatment episodes. In our experience we have seen patients who have failed large numbers of medication trials but respond extremely well to rTMS. We have also seen patients respond following a failed course of ECT, something that we thought initially was unlikely to be the case. The mechanisms of action of rTMS and ECT are likely to vary significantly, and at this stage there is no indication of any degree of overlap in the patients likely to respond to either treatment. Therefore, a course of rTMS should still be considered, especially as once patients have failed ECT they have few other treatment options.

It is also inevitable that as rTMS has become increasingly available, questions have arisen as to whether it should be presented as a first-line treatment option. To date, no substantive comparative data has been obtained as to the relative efficacy, or the efficacy compared to sham, in this early population. However, some studies have explored the use of rTMS in this population. In 2019 Voigt et al. undertook a systematic review to identify studies that had evaluated rTMS treatment in patients with depression who had failed to respond to one or fewer medication trials [8]. They identified six studies that were graded as high-quality (and four of lesser quality) and concluded that these provided good evidence that rTMS was effective in this early stage of the treatment course. Although this is an important finding, funding and clinical approval for rTMS treatment remains for patients in the more treatment-resistant phases of the illness in most places. In addition, the additional cost and complexity of rTMS treatment as compared to taking medication means that is likely to be a second-line therapy for most patients going forward. However, there is a significant percentage of the population who are resistant to the idea of taking medication for the treatment of depression, and for some of these patients, rTMS may be an attractive initial treatment option. In addition, it is possible to speculate that early intervention with a non-medication treatment such as rTMS may avoid medication-related complications and enhance brain plasticity in a way that ultimately improves long-term outcomes for patients with depression.

5.1.1 Clinical Recommendations

It appears reasonable for rTMS to be available as an option to patients with varying degrees of failure to respond to antidepressant strategies. However, response rates are likely to be higher in patients with lesser degrees of treatment resistance. It is possible that earlier intervention with rTMS may enhance longer-term outcomes, but further research, particularly focused on medication naive subjects, is required to establish this.

5.2 Illness Type: Unipolar and Bipolar Depression

Most clinical trials investigating the effectiveness of rTMS have predominately or exclusively enrolled patients with unipolar major depressive disorder. For example, the two largest multisite sham-controlled rTMS studies conducted to date excluded patients with bipolar disorder [9, 10]. Some studies, however, have included both patients in the depressive phase of bipolar disorder and those with unipolar depression. Within these trials, no analyses have suggested that a bipolar diagnosis is a negative predictor of the likelihood of clinical response. In one study of low-frequency stimulation applied to the right prefrontal cortex, patients with bipolar disorder had a substantially higher response rate (almost 70%) than the overall group (51%) [7]. However, most studies do not provide this sort of separate analysis to allow sufficient inferences to be made about the relative efficacy of rTMS subtypes in bipolar disorder. There is also a considerable lack of studies that have directly explored the antidepressant efficacy of rTMS in bipolar disorder alone.

In the first of these few studies, 20 patients were randomized to active or sham stimulation provided over 20 treatment sessions [11]. There was a significant improvement in depression with active but not sham stimulation. A second small study enrolled 23 patients and provided 5 Hz stimulation to the left DLPFC but failed to find a significant benefit of active stimulation over sham [12]. A third study, this time open-label, provided low-frequency stimulation applied to the right DLPFC [13]. Six of 11 patients responded and 4 achieved remission. A number of the patients with a greater degree of response remained well over a 12-month follow-up [14]. A more recent study included 19 patients with bipolar disorder who received open-label active rTMS using a novel coil providing deeper brain stimulation [15]. A significant improvement in depression was seen with a response rate greater than 60%. Of note, one patient experienced a generalized seizure during this trial. Despite these initial positive reports, there have been some negative randomized controlled trials (e.g., [16]), and the clinical trial evidence supporting the use of TMS in the treatment of bipolar depression cannot be considered definitive. A recent systematic review and meta-analysis identified 11 randomized sham-controlled trials with a total of 345 patients [17]. This analysis identified a small but significant improvement in depression scores and a greater rate of induction of remission with TMS than with sham although the analysis looking at response rates did not reach significance.

A number of reports have described switching to mania in patients receiving rTMS treatment for bipolar depression (e.g., [18–21]). However, the overall risk of this appears to be low and potentially no higher than that seen with sham stimulation [22]. No studies have systematically investigated whether the co-prescription of mood stabilizers reduces the possibility of a manic switch. However, in the absence of evidence that these medications can affect the efficacy of rTMS treatment, provision of mood stabilizing medication would be sensible in any patients who have previously experienced substantial manic symptoms. This would particularly include patients whose past symptoms required hospitalization or resulted in significant risks to the individual or others. The degree to which the patient can be monitored throughout the treatment course should also be taken into consideration. rTMS treatment should be withheld when manic symptoms are first evident during a course of treatment or when there is a dramatic shift in the level of mood symptoms.

Early research did investigate the possible treatment of mania with rTMS. In a small early study, manic symptoms appeared to be preferentially reduced with the provision of high-frequency rTMS to the right DLPFC compared to the left DLPFC [23]. Two subsequent case series showed promising results with high-frequency right-sided stimulation [24, 25], but when right DLPFC rTMS was completed to sham stimulation, no differences were seen [26]. More recently, and in contrast to this earlier research, a larger sham-controlled study of 41 patients has shown a substantial anti-manic effect of high-frequency right-sided stimulation [27]. Considerable further research is likely to be required before rTMS is considered a treatment for mania.

5.2.1 Clinical Recommendations

The vast majority of rTMS research has focused on the treatment of unipolar major depression. However, there is reasonable support at this stage for the use of rTMS in the treatment of patients with bipolar depression, especially given the clinical challenges with the management of this condition. The use of concurrent mood stabilizer medication should be carefully considered in patients with a history of substantial manic episodes and all patients monitored for the emergence of manic symptoms during treatment. The use of rTMS to treat mania is an area that requires further research before conclusions can be drawn on its clinical utility.

5.3 Elderly Patients with Depression

Depression, and especially treatment resistance, is clearly an important issue in the elderly [28]. Treatment resistance is more common in elderly patients with depression, and there are increasing complications with the use of other antidepressant modalities, including drug to drug interactions [29]. Views generally about the use of TMS in the elderly have evolved over time, from a belief that TMS was likely to be less, or ineffective, to the idea that TMS can safely and effectively be used in elderly patients with depression. The initial notion that TMS may be ineffective was drawn, in part, from two small and relatively under-powered or under-dosed clinical studies. First, a small randomized trial specifically conducted in elderly subjects (mean age 60 years) failed to show differences between active and sham stimulation [30]. However, treatment was only provided for 5 days and, based on pulse number and intensity, at very low dose. A second small trial provided treatment for 10 days but again at relatively low dose and in a small sample of only 24 patients. No differences between active and sham stimulation were found [31]. However, there were some positive outcomes in early reports. For example, in one study 49 elderly patients (mean age 69 years) received left- or right-sided rTMS. Treatment dose was quite variable and sometimes low (in some patients at 80% of the RMT) [32]. However, there was a significant overall reduction in depression symptoms and nine patients achieved response criteria.

Based on this initial conclusion that elderly patients may not respond to rTMS to the same degree, it was hypothesized that compared with younger patients, the elderly have a greater scalp to cortex distance in frontal areas relative to motor cortex. This would result in a lower degree of magnetic stimulus penetration resulting in poor clinical outcomes. One approach developed to address this involves the measurement of scalp to cortex distance on MRI scanning in DLPFC and motor cortex. An adjustment of stimulus intensity would then be made to take into account differences in motor cortex and frontal cortex scalp to cortex distance. Nahas et al. investigated this approach in 18 treatment-resistant elderly subjects (mean age 61 years) [33]. The applied intensities ranged up to 141% of the RMT. Five of the 18 patients responded to the adjusted treatment, but no comparison was made with non-adjusted rTMS. In an open-label trial, 6 out of 20 patients (mean age 66.8 years) responded to 2 weeks of treatment [34].

It is quite possible, however, that these initial negative reports have to do with study characteristics including sample size, dosing, and stimulus intensity. Differences in scalp to cortex distance may well be important if stimulation is being applied at subthreshold intensities (e.g., at less than 100% of the RMT) but may be much less important when stimulation is applied at higher intensities which is now more commonly the case. Over time, information on the use of TMS in the elderly has progressively become more positive. For example, in the analysis of the effect of age in larger treatment samples, it has increasingly been seen as not being relevant to antidepressant response. For example, in several large studies we have conducted, there has been no relationship evident between age and a poorer response to rTMS treatment (e.g., [7, 35]). In a recent open-label study of 130 patients treated in a naturalistic setting, there was also no relationship found between clinical response and age [36]. One of the largest explorations of demographic predictors of response to treatment actually found that older age was a positive predictor of outcome [37] and there was no association between age and response in the large 5000+ patient study of Sackeim et al. [38]. In addition, a greater response rate in elderly subjects than young subjects was found in a recent study of twice-daily rTMS [39], and a second recent study showed a significant difference over sham stimulation of dTMS in an elderly group [40].

Anecdotally, we have treated patients with depression across the elderly spectrum including patients in their late 80s and early 90s. Treatment has been well tolerated, with no substantial difference in patient experiences or response compared with younger subjects.

5.3.1 Clinical Recommendations

Treatment-resistant depression in the elderly is common and other treatment alternatives can be frequently difficult to administer. rTMS should be considered as a treatment option in this age group provided with confidence that substantive antidepressant response rates are likely to be achieved.

5.4 Adolescent Depression

A quite limited literature has explored the potential use of rTMS in the treatment of depression in adolescents. The first published paper described the treatment of three adolescent patients and four 18-year-olds with 2 weeks of high-frequency stimulation applied to the left DLPFC [41]. A relatively low dose of stimulation was used (1600 pulses per session). Two of the three adolescent patients improved with treatment. A subsequent report evaluated treatment efficacy in two adolescent patients provided with a slightly higher dose of rTMS treatment (2000 pulses per day) with clinical response seen in both patients [42]. A third case series included five subjects younger than 18 [43]. Each patient received 14 treatment sessions (400 pulses per session). Three of the five patients had a significant reduction in depressive symptoms. No major adverse events were reported in any of the patients described in this case series.

A recent systematic review identified 18 open-label studies with a total of 142 treated patients [44]. Antidepressant effects were generally reported across these studies but there were no significant sham-controlled trials identified. In one interesting report of open-label treatment, response rates in adolescents were higher than those in patients from older age groups [45].

In regard to safety, a report described the development of a generalized seizure in a 16-year-old female patient during the first session of a planned course of rTMS treatment [46]. The patient had no predisposing factors for the development of a seizure, but was receiving 100 mg of sertraline per day at the time. The authors of this case report do not describe a clear progression of tonic clonic activity and it is possible that the event was a syncopal seizure. Notably, the dose of rTMS provided in this case was quite low (4-s 10 Hz trains at 80% of the motor threshold). It has been proposed that the seizure threshold may be lower in this age group, extrapolating from the situation with ECT [47]. However, this has not been systematically studied. Over 1000 subjects under 18 have received single or paired pulse TMS in investigative studies without the report of any seizures [48].

It is worth noting that two adolescents receiving TMS in a stroke study were reported to have experienced a syncopal event [49], and practitioners should be aware of this possibility, especially where there is a history of syncope with other procedures such as injections. In our experience, pre-syncopal activity (feeling faint) is much common with TMS in young people and especially in those who have fainted or become syncopal with injections or other medical procedures.

5.4.1 Clinical Recommendations

Limited systematic research has explored the use of rTMS in the treatment of depression in adolescents. Practitioners should be aware of the possibility of syncope and potentially a lower seizure threshold. rTMS presents as a potentially promising way to avoid the early use of medication treatments but should not be adopted clinically until evaluated adequately.

5.5 Pregnant or Breastfeeding Patients

The presentation of patients with depression in the antenatal or postnatal period often poses significant management challenges. There are frequently concerns about the potential impact of antidepressant medications during these periods, and ECT is often avoided during pregnancy due to concerns about the anesthetic and the seizure itself. Given that the magnetic field produced with a TMS device is very localized, it is unlikely that a fetus would experience significant exposure to a substantial magnetic field if rTMS was applied during pregnancy. In fact, electrical fuel modeling suggests that there should be no meaningful exposure to the magnetic field in the fetus [50] although it is possible that the noise produced by the TMS device could impact the developing auditory system. There are clearly no child safety issues with postnatal rTMS provision. As such, rTMS treatment appeals as an alternative option for the treatment of depression presenting in the antenatal and postnatal periods. However, limited research to date has explored the use of rTMS applied at these times, and the rTMS option should be evaluated carefully for each individual.

In regard to pregnancy, a number of case reports have been published since 1999, with no evidence of major adverse events (e.g., [51]) and one early report described a case series of ten patients treated during the second or third trimester [52]. These patients received low-frequency right-sided rTMS in up to 20 treatment sessions with 7 experiencing clinical response. No adverse maternal or fetal outcomes emerged. A more recent follow-up study of children born from mothers who were treated during pregnancy found some language developmental delays, but these were no different to those found in children of mothers with depression untreated with rTMS [53]. Kim et al. recently published the results of a small randomized study of 1 Hz right-sided rTMS in pregnant women in the second or third term of pregnancy [54]. A greater degree of reduction in depression was seen with active compared to sham treatment. There were three late preterm births in the active treatment group (two of these mothers had other risk factors for preterm delivery) but no other adverse maternal and delivery-related outcomes.

One study explored the potential acceptability of rTMS treatment to pregnant women [55]. Researchers surveyed 500 pregnant women and a second sample of 51 women who were exposed to an educational video providing information about rTMS treatment. rTMS was not considered acceptable in the first study, but was considered acceptable by 15.7% of the second sample after provision of the information video.

A similarly narrow range of research has explored the use of rTMS in postpartum depression. One case report described the use of rTMS in the successful postpartum management of a patient with bipolar disorder where rTMS was used for the treatment of both mania and depression [56]. One case series has described the management of nine antidepressant-free women with postpartum depression treated with high-frequency left DLPFC rTMS over 4 weeks [57]. Eight patients achieved remission of depression during acute treatment. Seven of these remained in remission after 6 months without further psychiatric treatment. The only randomized trial included only 14 patients and found significant benefits of active over sham stimulation despite the small sample size [58]. An open-label study included 25 patients, of whom 14 achieved remission but of note 6 patients dropped out because of scheduling or access issues [59]. Clearly attending for rTMS on a daily basis is likely to be complicated for mothers in the very early postpartum period.

Despite these promising initial findings, rTMS treatment in pregnancy or the postpartum period should proceed cautiously. Although it is unlikely that an unborn fetus would be exposed to substantial magnetic fields, it is possible that hormonal changes induced by rTMS could have adverse effects and this will require systematic research. rTMS could also induce changes in the hormonal profile of breast milk. In addition, provision of rTMS during pregnancy may require the more careful monitoring of motor thresholds and rTMS dose as hormonal fluctuations may affect cortical excitability over time.

5.5.1 Clinical Recommendations

Limited research has evaluated the use of rTMS in pregnancy or the postpartum period, to date. However, there are strong reasons to avoid other biological treatments during these times. This is likely to lead to the consideration of the use of rTMS in spite of the limited evidence available for its use. Provision of rTMS under these circumstances should include a careful assessment of the risks and potential benefits of both rTMS and other treatment alternatives. Further research is clearly required in this area.

5.6 Comorbid Anxiety

Anxiety symptoms are extremely common in patients with major depressive disorder, and there is a high rate of comorbidity between depression and primary anxiety disorders themselves. As such, patients will very frequently present for the treatment of depression with rTMS who have substantial ongoing anxiety. What we can advise patient under these circumstances is informed by studies in patients primarily with depression, but also a small range of studies that have explored the use of rTMS in the treatment of anxiety disorders themselves. This latter literature suggests that TMS might have efficacy in the primary treatment of anxiety although the studies are few (e.g., [60]). A greater number of studies demonstrating anti-anxiety effects with rTMS have been conducted with low-frequency right-sided rTMS although this is not ubiquitous.

In regard to the response of anxiety symptoms when treating MDD, the largest study (over 1100 patients) exploring the effect of a concurrent anxiety disorder comorbidity on antidepressant responses found that patients with a comorbid anxiety disorder had a lower rate of response than those without, although patients with an anxiety disorder still had a substantial response rate [37]. The response rate varied from 35% for patients with panic disorder to 47% for generalized anxiety disorder and 48% for PTSD. A second study, somewhat smaller study, of 248 patients found no differences in outcomes for patients with comorbid anxiety disorder [61].

5.6.1 Clinical Recommendations

The presence of comorbid anxiety should not be a reason to hold back TMS treatment for depression and there is a reasonably expectation that anxiety symptoms will improve with successful rTMS therapy.

5.7 Depression with Psychotic Symptoms

There is little research on which to base recommendations in regard to the likelihood of efficacy of rTMS treatment in patients with depression with psychotic symptoms. Patients with psychotic symptoms have been excluded from almost all TMS clinical trials conducted since the early 2000s. This is likely to have occurred in response to the results of an early rTMS study published in 2000 [62]. In this study, one of the first that compared antidepressant effects of rTMS to ECT, nine patients with psychotic symptoms who received rTMS had a lesser antidepressant effects than those ten who received ECT.

It is notable, however, that the rTMS dose was only 400 pulses per day and a total of 20 treatments all applied at 90% of the RMT. Interestingly, the ECT group received an unlimited number of unilateral bilateral ECT. The lack of equality between the treatment groups and the extremely low dose of rTMS makes the comparison fairly meaningless in the context of modern methods of TMS delivery, but unfortunately the results of this study seemed to have effectively stifled the investigation of the use of rTMS in this clinical group.

Since 2000, several other ECT-rTMS trials have included some psychotic patients but very small numbers. In a small meta-analysis ECT appeared to be more effective than rTMS in the studies with mixed samples (although not more effective in non-psychotic samples), but the total data was less than 60 subjects and not a single one of these trials used TMS at 120% of the RMT or for more than 20 sessions [63].

5.7.1 Clinical Recommendations

rTMS has not been shown to be ineffective in patients with psychotic symptoms, but unfortunately, we really have no meaningful data on whether it is actually clinically effective. As such patients with psychotic symptoms should be offered effective therapy such as ECT and rTMS only provided in the context of clinical research.

5.8 Concurrent Illness: Neurological Disease

A small literature has begun to explore whether rTMS is safe and has efficacy in the treatment of patients with depression in the context of substantive comorbid neurological conditions. Depression is a commonly occurring comorbidity in several neurological illnesses. For example, depression is common in the context of development and persistence of Parkinson's disease [64]. In the first rTMS study to address this clinical group, Dragasevic et al. provided low-frequency frontal rTMS to ten depressed subjects producing a significant reduction in depression despite a low dose of stimulation. A second open study also reported a significant reduction in depression, this time with high-frequency stimulation applied in 14 patients [65]. A small ($n = 22$), sham-controlled study of 5 Hz prefrontal DLPFC rTMS also supported the antidepressant effects of rTMS in depression in patients with Parkinson's disease [66].

In a similar manner, open-label data has been collected on the use of rTMS in the treatment of vascular depression or depression that presented following stroke. Jorge et al. randomized 92 patients with depression and substantive vascular disease to active or sham left DLPFC rTMS [67]. Substantial antidepressant effects were seen with active treatment in two dose groups compared to sham. In the first trial in post-stroke depression, antidepressant effects greater than sham were seen in a small group of patients receiving 10 Hz stimulation to the left DLPFC [68]. These findings were confirmed in a subsequent double-blind study, which compared 1 Hz rTMS, 10 Hz rTMS, and sham stimulation in patients with post-stroke depression [69]. High-frequency stimulation resulted in improved depression scores although no cognitive improvements were evident.

A third condition that is beginning to be explored is the presentation of depression subsequent to a brain injury. This appears to be a relatively common occurrence but a history of traumatic head injury has frequently been an exclusion criterion in rTMS treatment trials. Several small trials have now been published following an initial case report described promising early results [70]. We found no significant antidepressant benefits in a small study of sequential bilateral rTMS applied for patients with depression post-traumatic brain injury [71], but some more promising results have also been reported (see systematic review in [72]).

5.8.1 Clinical Recommendations

The presence of an underlying or comorbid neurological disease such as stroke or Parkinson's disease does not appear to prevent the possibility of successful response to rTMS treatment. The use of rTMS treatment under these circumstances should be balanced against any potential increased risks of seizure induction related to the underlying disease entity with substantial potential benefits if clinical response is achieved.

5.9 Other Factors

There are a number of other factors that may influence the likelihood of a successful course of rTMS treatment. There are clearly some individuals who for physiological personality reasons are substantially more sensitive to pain or discomfort and will struggle to tolerate a course of rTMS treatment. Likewise, there are individuals who are more likely to experience headaches resulting from rTMS treatment and had difficulty tolerating this. These issues are probably more likely in patients with a history of significant pain problems, and caution should be taken when initiating treatment in individuals with a history of substantial preexisting headaches. In individuals like this, a slowly increasing stimulus intensity should be considered and low-frequency right-sided rTMS may be a sensible treatment option.

Preexisting neck pain can also complicate a course of rTMS treatment. Patients are required to sit still for a significant period of time, and unless the neck is adequately supported, this may lead to significant discomfort. Under these circumstances, care should be taken to ensure that the patient is in a comfortable position at all times. The patient may need to have brief breaks during each treatment session to minimize the development of muscle spasm.

The presence of significant psychiatric comorbidity may also limit the likelihood of treatment response although this has not been systematically evaluated in many studies. In our clinical experience, comorbid anxiety symptoms may improve with the successful resolution of depression treated with rTMS, but this is not always the case. When anxiety symptoms persist, this is likely to have a long-term negative impact on the patient's mood and contribute to earlier depressive relapse. In our experience, comorbid obsessive-compulsive symptoms are rarely successfully alleviated with standard rTMS depression protocols.

Clinical Considerations in Patient Selection and Recommendations

- rTMS may be effective in patients with a wide range of degrees of treatment resistance. It is a reasonable option in patients who have failed one or more antidepressant medication therapies.
- rTMS should not be withheld because of a concern that patients have too great a degree of treatment resistance.
- rTMS has established efficacy in unipolar depression.
- There is considerably less evidence for the efficacy of rTMS in bipolar depression. However, given the challenges with treating this condition, the provision of rTMS therapy can be justified given the evidence collected to date.
- In patients with bipolar affective disorder, especially type I, concurrent mood stabilization should be utilized to prevent manic switching.
- rTMS treatment of depression is effective and safe in the elderly.
- rTMS treatment of depression remains experimental in children and adolescents.
- The limited data so far suggests that rTMS treatment is safe in pregnancy and during breastfeeding, but considerably greater treatment numbers are required to establish safety with any degree of certainty in these groups.
- There is a reasonable likelihood that patients with comorbid anxiety will experience a reduction in anxiety symptoms during treatment of MDD regardless of the choice of rTMS stimulation approach.
- Clinical trials have not adequately explored whether rTMS can be used in the treatment of patients with depression with psychotic symptoms.
- Patients may be able to be successfully and safely treated for depression when they have comorbid neurological disorders such as Parkinson's disease or vascular cognitive changes. Epilepsy, however, remains a contraindication to the use of rTMS.

References

1. Fava M (2003) Diagnosis and definition of treatment-resistant depression. Biol Psychiatry 53(8):649–659
2. Sackeim HA (2016) Acute continuation and maintenance treatment of major depressive episodes with transcranial magnetic stimulation. Brain Stimul 9(3):313–319
3. Ruhe HG et al (2012) Staging methods for treatment resistant depression. A systematic review. J Affect Disord 137(1–3):35–45
4. Sackeim HA et al (1990) The impact of medication resistance and continuation pharmacotherapy on relapse following response to electroconvulsive therapy in major depression. J Clin Psychopharmacol 10(2):96–104
5. Lisanby SH et al (2009) Daily left prefrontal repetitive transcranial magnetic stimulation in the acute treatment of major depression: clinical predictors of outcome in a multisite, randomized controlled clinical trial. Neuropsychopharmacology 34(2):522–534

6. Fregni F et al (2006) Predictors of antidepressant response in clinical trials of transcranial magnetic stimulation. Int J Neuropsychopharmacol 9(6):641–654
7. Fitzgerald PB et al (2006) A randomized trial of low-frequency right-prefrontal-cortex transcranial magnetic stimulation as augmentation in treatment-resistant major depression. Int J Neuropsychopharmacol 9(6):655–666
8. Voigt J, Carpenter L, Leuchter A (2019) A systematic literature review of the clinical efficacy of repetitive transcranial magnetic stimulation (rTMS) in non-treatment resistant patients with major depressive disorder. BMC Psychiatry 19(1):13
9. George MS et al (2010) Daily left prefrontal transcranial magnetic stimulation therapy for major depressive disorder: a sham-controlled randomized trial. Arch Gen Psychiatry 67(5):507–516
10. O'Reardon JP et al (2007) Efficacy and safety of transcranial magnetic stimulation in the acute treatment of major depression: a multisite randomized controlled trial. Biol Psychiatry 62(11):1208–1216
11. Dolberg OT et al (2002) Transcranial magnetic stimulation in patients with bipolar depression: a double blind, controlled study. Bipolar Disord 4(Suppl 1):94–95
12. Nahas Z et al (2003) Left prefrontal transcranial magnetic stimulation (TMS) treatment of depression in bipolar affective disorder: a pilot study of acute safety and efficacy. Bipolar Disord 5(1):40–47
13. Dell'Osso B et al (2009) Augmentative repetitive navigated transcranial magnetic stimulation (rTMS) in drug-resistant bipolar depression. Bipolar Disord 11(1):76–81
14. Dell'Osso B et al (2011) Long-term efficacy after acute augmentative repetitive transcranial magnetic stimulation in bipolar depression: a 1-year follow-up study. J ECT 27(2):141–144
15. Harel EV et al (2011) H-coil repetitive transcranial magnetic stimulation for the treatment of bipolar depression: an add-on, safety and feasibility study. World J Biol Psychiatry 12(2):119–126
16. Fitzgerald PB et al (2016) A negative double-blind controlled trial of sequential bilateral rTMS in the treatment of bipolar depression. J Affect Disord 198:158–162
17. Tee MMK, Au CH (2020) A systematic review and meta-analysis of randomized sham-controlled trials of repetitive transcranial magnetic stimulation for bipolar disorder. Psychiatry Q 91(4):1225–1247
18. Garcia-Toro M (1999) Acute manic symptomatology during repetitive transcranial magnetic stimulation in a patient with bipolar depression. Br J Psychiatry 175:491
19. Hausmann A et al (2004) Can bilateral prefrontal repetitive transcranial magnetic stimulation (rTMS) induce mania? A case report. J Clin Psychiatry 65(11):1575–1576
20. Huang CC, Su TP, Shan IK (2004) A case report of repetitive transcranial magnetic stimulation-induced mania. Bipolar Disord 6(5):444–445
21. Sakkas P et al (2003) Induction of mania by rTMS: report of two cases. Eur Psychiatry 18(4):196–198
22. Xia G et al (2008) Treatment-emergent mania in unipolar and bipolar depression: focus on repetitive transcranial magnetic stimulation. Int J Neuropsychopharmacol 11(1):119–130
23. Grisaru N et al (1998) Transcranial magnetic stimulation in mania: a controlled study. Am J Psychiatry 155(11):1608–1610
24. Saba G et al (2004) Repetitive transcranial magnetic stimulation as an add-on therapy in the treatment of mania: a case series of eight patients. Psychiatry Res 128(2):199–202
25. Michael N, Erfurth A (2004) Treatment of bipolar mania with right prefrontal rapid transcranial magnetic stimulation. J Affect Disord 78(3):253–257
26. Kaptsan A et al (2003) Right prefrontal TMS versus sham treatment of mania: a controlled study. Bipolar Disord 5(1):36–39
27. Praharaj SK, Ram D, Arora M (2009) Efficacy of high frequency (rapid) suprathreshold repetitive transcranial magnetic stimulation of right prefrontal cortex in bipolar mania: a randomized sham controlled study. J Affect Disord 117(3):146–150
28. Bonner D, Howard R (1995) Treatment-resistant depression in the elderly. Int Psychogeriatr 7(Suppl):83–94

29. Baldwin RC, Simpson S (1997) Treatment resistant depression in the elderly: a review of its conceptualisation, management and relationship to organic brain disease. J Affect Disord 46(3):163–173
30. Manes F et al (2001) A controlled study of repetitive transcranial magnetic stimulation as a treatment of depression in the elderly. Int Psychogeriatr 13(2):225–231
31. Mosimann UP et al (2004) Repetitive transcranial magnetic stimulation: a putative add-on treatment for major depression in elderly patients. Psychiatry Res 126(2):123–133
32. Milev R et al (2009) Repetitive transcranial magnetic stimulation for treatment of medication-resistant depression in older adults: a case series. J ECT 25(1):44–49
33. Nahas Z et al (2004) Safety and benefits of distance-adjusted prefrontal transcranial magnetic stimulation in depressed patients 55–75 years of age: a pilot study. Depress Anxiety 19(4):249–256
34. Abraham G et al (2007) Repetitive transcranial magnetic stimulation for treatment of elderly patients with depression - an open label trial. Neuropsychiatr Dis Treat 3(6):919–924
35. Fitzgerald PB et al (2010) A randomized trial of unilateral and bilateral prefrontal cortex transcranial magnetic stimulation in treatment-resistant major depression. Psychol Med 41(6):1187–1196
36. Frank E et al (2011) Transcranial magnetic stimulation for the treatment of depression: feasibility and results under naturalistic conditions: a retrospective analysis. Eur Arch Psychiatry Clin Neurosci 261(4):261–266
37. Fitzgerald PB et al (2016) A study of the pattern of response to rTMS treatment in depression. Depress Anxiety 33(8):746–753
38. Sackeim HA et al (2020) Clinical outcomes in a large registry of patients with major depressive disorder treated with transcranial magnetic stimulation. J Affect Disord 277:65–74
39. Desbeaumes Jodoin V, Miron JP, Lesperance P (2019) Safety and efficacy of accelerated repetitive transcranial magnetic stimulation protocol in elderly depressed unipolar and bipolar patients. Am J Geriatr Psychiatry 27(5):548–558
40. Kaster TS et al (2018) Efficacy, tolerability, and cognitive effects of deep transcranial magnetic stimulation for late-life depression: a prospective randomized controlled trial. Neuropsychopharmacology 43(11):2231–2238
41. Walter G et al (2001) Transcranial magnetic stimulation in young persons: a review of known cases. J Child Adolesc Psychopharmacol 11(1):69–75
42. Loo C, McFarquhar T, Walter G (2006) Transcranial magnetic stimulation in adolescent depression. Australas Psychiatry 14(1):81–85
43. Bloch Y et al (2008) Repetitive transcranial magnetic stimulation in the treatment of depression in adolescents: an open-label study. J ECT 24(2):156–159
44. Hett D et al (2021) Repetitive transcranial magnetic stimulation (rTMS) for the treatment of depression in adolescence: a systematic review. J Affect Disord 278:460–469
45. Zhang T et al (2019) Add-on rTMS for the acute treatment of depressive symptoms is probably more effective in adolescents than in adults: evidence from real-world clinical practice. Brain Stimul 12(1):103–109
46. Hu SH et al (2011) Repetitive transcranial magnetic stimulation-induced seizure of a patient with adolescent-onset depression: a case report and literature review. J Int Med Res 39(5):2039–2044
47. D'Agati D et al (2010) rTMS for adolescents: safety and efficacy considerations. Psychiatry Res 177(3):280–285
48. Quintana H (2005) Transcranial magnetic stimulation in persons younger than the age of 18. J ECT 21(2):88–95
49. Kirton A et al (2008) Neurocardiogenic syncope complicating pediatric transcranial magnetic stimulation. Pediatr Neurol 39(3):196–197
50. Yanamadala J et al (2017) Estimates of peak electric fields induced by transcranial magnetic stimulation in pregnant women as patients using an FEM full-body model. Conf Proc IEEE Eng Med Biol Soc 2017:1441–1444

51. Nahas Z et al (1999) Safety and feasibility of repetitive transcranial magnetic stimulation in the treatment of anxious depression in pregnancy: a case report. J Clin Psychiatry 60(1):50–52
52. Kim DR et al (2011) An open label pilot study of transcranial magnetic stimulation for pregnant women with major depressive disorder. J Womens Health (Larchmt) 20(2):255–261
53. Eryilmaz G et al (2015) Follow-up study of children whose mothers were treated with transcranial magnetic stimulation during pregnancy: preliminary results. Neuromodulation 18(4):255–260
54. Kim DR et al (2019) Randomized controlled trial of transcranial magnetic stimulation in pregnant women with major depressive disorder. Brain Stimul 12(1):96–102
55. Kim DR et al (2011) A survey of patient acceptability of repetitive transcranial magnetic stimulation (TMS) during pregnancy. J Affect Disord 129(1–3):385–390
56. Cohen RB et al (2008) Use of repetitive transcranial magnetic stimulation for the management of bipolar disorder during the postpartum period. Brain Stimul 1(3):224–226
57. Garcia KS et al (2010) Repetitive transcranial magnetic stimulation treats postpartum depression. Brain Stimul 3(1):36–41
58. Myczkowski ML et al (2012) Effects of repetitive transcranial magnetic stimulation on clinical, social, and cognitive performance in postpartum depression. Neuropsychiatr Dis Treat 8:491–500
59. Brock DG et al (2016) Effectiveness of NeuroStar transcranial magnetic stimulation (TMS) in patients with major depressive disorder with postpartum onset. Brain Stimul 9(5):e7
60. Diefenbach GJ et al (2016) Repetitive transcranial magnetic stimulation for generalised anxiety disorder: a pilot randomised, double-blind, sham-controlled trial. Br J Psychiatry 209(3):222–228
61. Clarke E et al (2019) Efficacy of repetitive transcranial magnetic stimulation in the treatment of depression with comorbid anxiety disorders. J Affect Disord 252:435–439
62. Grunhaus L et al (2000) Repetitive transcranial magnetic stimulation is as effective as electroconvulsive therapy in the treatment of nondelusional major depressive disorder: an open study. Biol Psychiatry 47(4):314–324
63. Ren J et al (2014) Repetitive transcranial magnetic stimulation versus electroconvulsive therapy for major depression: a systematic review and meta-analysis. Prog Neuropsychopharmacol Biol Psychiatry 51:181–189
64. Reijnders JS et al (2008) A systematic review of prevalence studies of depression in Parkinson's disease. Mov Disord 23(2):183–189. quiz 313
65. Epstein CM et al (2007) An open study of repetitive transcranial magnetic stimulation in treatment-resistant depression with Parkinson's disease. Clin Neurophysiol 118(10):2189–2194
66. Pal E et al (2010) The impact of left prefrontal repetitive transcranial magnetic stimulation on depression in Parkinson's disease: a randomized, double-blind, placebo-controlled study. Mov Disord 25(14):2311–2317
67. Jorge RE et al (2008) Treatment of vascular depression using repetitive transcranial magnetic stimulation. Arch Gen Psychiatry 65(3):268–276
68. Jorge RE et al (2004) Repetitive transcranial magnetic stimulation as treatment of poststroke depression: a preliminary study. Biol Psychiatry 55(4):398–405
69. Kim BR et al (2010) Effect of repetitive transcranial magnetic stimulation on cognition and mood in stroke patients: a double-blind, sham-controlled trial. Am J Phys Med Rehabil 89(5):362–368
70. Fitzgerald PB et al (2010) Transcranial magnetic stimulation for depression following traumatic brain injury: a case study. J ECT 27(1):38–40
71. Hoy KE et al (2019) A pilot investigation of repetitive transcranial magnetic stimulation for post-traumatic brain injury depression: safety, tolerability, and efficacy. J Neurotrauma 36(13):2092–2098
72. Beedham W et al (2020) The management of depression following traumatic brain injury: a systematic review with meta-analysis. Brain Inj 34(10):1287–1304

6 Practical Issues in Treatment Provision

Abstract

The provision of rTMS treatment requires the individual prescription of a variety of treatment parameters including the intensity of stimulation, its frequency, and the characteristics of the stimulation trains provided. The intensity of stimulation should be determined based on an assessment of an individual subjects' resting motor threshold in the hemisphere to which stimulation will be applied using one of a number of standard methods. Choice of individual stimulation parameters should be influenced by consideration of the literature establishing efficacy as well as individual patient factors such as stimulation tolerability. Most rTMS treatment courses are provided 5 days per week over a period of time extending somewhere between 4 and 6 weeks. There are several possible methods for localization of the TMS coil and the method chosen for this purpose may influence clinical efficacy. It is not necessary to withdraw patients from medication prior to commencing rTMS treatment although commencing new medication treatment during rTMS treatment may not be ideal.

6.1 Introduction

At the commencement of a treatment course, the prescribing practitioner is required to determine a variety of parameters for treatment provision. The choice of these should be made on an individual patient basis but may be influenced or largely determined by local policies or established protocols. Each of the following parameters must be explicitly prescribed for each patient or made clear in local protocols:

- Intensity of stimulation
- Frequency of stimulation
- Duration of each stimulation train

P. B. Fitzgerald, Z. J. Daskalakis, *rTMS Treatment for Depression*,
https://doi.org/10.1007/978-3-030-91519-3_6

- Total number of stimulation trains provided in each treatment session
- Intertrain interval
- Site of stimulation
- Coil orientation

Dosing issues in regard to the intensity of stimulation, especially in relation to the processes for assessing the resting motor threshold (RMT), are addressed in Chap. 12.

6.2 Selection of Treatment Type and Parameters

As discussed in Chap. 4, a considerable body of research has evaluated a variety of methods of rTMS application including high-frequency stimulation applied to the left DLPFC, low-frequency stimulation applied to the right DLPFC, and variations of bilateral stimulation. Clearly, the vast majority of research has established the efficacy of high-frequency stimulation applied to the left DLPFC, most commonly at 10 Hz. This data includes the pivotal Neuronetics Ltd.-sponsored clinical trial that led to device registration in the USA. As such, it is likely that high-frequency stimulation applied to the left DLPFC is likely to be the initial rTMS treatment option selected for most patients.

6.2.1 Considerations with High-Frequency Stimulation Left-Sided rTMS

Frequency: Although there are antidepressant studies of the effect of frequencies such as 5 and 20 Hz, the vast majority of studies have been conducted with 10 Hz stimulation. This includes the two main large randomized multisite rTMS trials [1, 2]. There are no studies showing any particular advantage of stimulation at other frequencies. Given the depth of research that has focused on this particular frequency, unless evidence emerges to the contrary, most treatment should be provided at 10 Hz.

Train Duration and Intensity: As discussed previously, there is a relationship between train duration and intensity in regard to the safety of rTMS administration. If trains are to be provided at an intensity of 120% of the RMT, train duration should be limited to 4.2 s. Longer trains, most commonly 5 s in duration, can be safely administered at lower intensity, for example, 110% of the RMT.

Train Number: 75 trains of 10 Hz stimulation were applied in the two large multisite rTMS trials conducted to date [1, 2]. This was considerably in excess of the number of trains used in most trials until that time, with previous studies often applying only 20–30 trains. Given that the remission rates in both of these trials were fairly modest, it is not clear whether this increase in train number resulted in substantially greater efficacy than had been seen previously. In a large recent study exploring train number, we found no greater antidepressant effects using 125 trains in a single session compared to 50 trains [3]. This suggests that at 75 trains we are likely to be at the top of the dose response curve, and within an individual stimulation session, there is probably little value in providing a greater number. As such, 75 trains per treatment session are likely to remain the de facto standard treatment going forward.

Intertrain Interval: Although historically high-frequency 10 Hz rTMS has been administered with a relatively long train interval, most commonly 26 s, when a 4-s train of stimulation is applied, evidence has emerged that it is safe and appropriate to reduce this duration to potentially reduce the overall length of left-sided treatment. We found no adverse consequences of decreasing to a 15-s train interval in 150 patients receiving 10 Hz treatment [3], and Neuronetics have received FDA approval for a protocol with an 11-s interval. A recent study compared the outcomes of 1493 patients treated with this "Dash" protocol with those achieved in 613 patients who receive treatment with a 25-s interval with data taken from real-world treatment recorded through registry [4]. There were no differences in clinical outcomes achieved between these two schedules. The article reporting this data also indicated that Neuronetics had not received increasing rates of reports of seizures since clearance of the Dash protocol. Rates of other side effects such as headache and scalp pain were not reported but presumably may be slightly higher in patients treated more intensively.

6.2.2 Use of Low-Frequency Right-Sided rTMS

There are a number of potential advantages of low-frequency right-sided rTMS that could lead to its potential consideration as a first-line treatment or, alternatively, as an approach in circumstances where high-frequency stimulation cannot be tolerated or may be considered potentially unsafe. Low-frequency stimulation, especially as it is known to reduce cortical excitability rather than increase cortical excitability, is likely to be associated with a substantially lower risk of seizure induction. Therefore, there may be circumstances in which the risks associated with a trial of low-frequency stimulation may be considered appropriate, but high-frequency stimulation raises too high a risk of seizure induction. This could be because an individual patient has a risk factor for seizure induction or heightened cortical excitability. It could also be because the risk of actually experiencing a seizure may be considered too high, for example, in somebody with compromised cardiac function. It should be noted however, that the risk of seizure induction with low-frequency stimulation is not zero, but is likely to be less than with high-frequency stimulation.

Another circumstance in which low-frequency right-sided stimulation may be considered as an alternative is where high-frequency stimulation is not tolerated by individual subjects. The vast majority of patients will find low-frequency stimulation more tolerable than the intense bursts of high-frequency stimulation although this is not universal.

Finally, right-sided stimulation may be considered as a treatment option in patients who have failed to respond to high-frequency left-sided rTMS. Studies which have compared the two approaches have generally found equivalent efficacy [5]. Little research has explored rates of response to one treatment in the event of failure of the other. We previously found that a minority of patients will respond to a trial of high-frequency left-sided rTMS if they had failed to respond to low-frequency right-sided rTMS. However, no systematic research has explored cross-over in the opposite direction. However, given the low risks associated with low-frequency right-sided stimulation, this could be considered a treatment alternative in some patients.

Dosing of Low-Frequency Right-Sided rTMS: Early studies of low-frequency right-sided rTMS applied a small number of 60 s trains, usually with a 30- or 60-s intertrain interval. More recent studies have commonly used a single 15- or 20-min train (900–1200 pulses) in each treatment session. This dosing remains much lower than the common dosing with 10 Hz stimulation (3750 pulses across 75 trains per session). We found no benefit of increasing the train duration length to 60 min compared to 20 min [3] and typically use a 20-min train and standard applications. Low-frequency right-sided stimulation is typically applied at 120% of the RMT.

6.2.3 Sequential Bilateral rTMS

Sequential bilateral TMS involving the application of both low-frequency right-sided and high-frequency left-sided rTMS was developed to investigate whether combining both of these effective antidepressant strategies into one treatment would result in a more effective approach. Initial trials of this approach were promising with substantial response and remission rates [6] and at least one study has found superior efficacy than unilateral treatment [7]. However, a number of other studies have found equivalent or inferior responses to bilateral compared to unilateral rTMS (e.g., [8–10]). When the research data exploring the use of sequential bilateral rTMS has been synthesized in meta-analyses, it appears to demonstrate clear efficacy compared to sham stimulation [11] but at a level which appears to be similar to that seen with unilateral rTMS [12]. Note one study has shown a greater reduction of suicidal ideation with bilateral compared to unilateral and sham stimulation and this certainly warrants replication [13].

Dosing of Low-Frequency Right-Sided rTMS: This typically involves a combination of a standard low-frequency right-sided rTMS train (20 min) and 50 or 75 trains of high-frequency left-sided 10 Hz stimulation, both applied at 120% of the RMT. The intertrain interval for left-sided treatment may be reduced (as above) to reduce the overall protocol time.

6.2.4 Overall Clinical Recommendations

At this stage under most circumstances, a first-line rTMS treatment is likely to entail 10 Hz stimulation applied to the left DLPFC. Under most circumstances, a dose of seventy-five 4-s trains applied at up 120% of the RMT is recommended. An intertrain interval of anywhere between 11 and 26 s would seem to be reasonable with no significant risks associated with a shorter duration. It is likely that many patients, especially those with an RMT of greater than 50%, will benefit from a progressive increase in treatment intensity over the course of one or more treatment sessions until the target dose is achieved. When practitioners measuring the RMT have limited experience, dosing at 110% of the RMT is sensible to ensure that there is a margin of safety in case of minor errors in RMT estimation. Low-frequency right-sided stimulation is a good option for patients who have trouble tolerating left-sided treatment and who have additional risk factors for seizure induction or when left-sided treatment has failed to produce therapeutic effects.

The role of sequential bilateral TMS remains unclear. One circumstance in which its use may be sensibly considered is in the treatment of a patient who has partially responded to an initial trial of unilateral treatment. If treatment response is inadequate but there has been benefit achieved, switching to bilateral treatment to continue the application of the initial paradigm while adding a new therapeutic intervention may be preferable from switching away from something which has been partially effective (see further discussion in Chap. 7).

6.3 Treatment Scheduling and Duration

6.3.1 Less Intense Approaches

The vast majority of rTMS studies have provided treatment 5 days per week, Monday to Friday, including the trials that have led to clinical approval, and as such this is very much the standard adopted in clinical practice for the use of rTMS therapy.

A small number of studies have investigated whether clinical responses can be achieved with less intensive treatment schedules. In the first study of this nature, a small group of patients were randomized to have treatment 5 days a week or to receive three treatments in week 1 and two treatments in week 2 [14]. There were no significant differences seen in outcomes between the two groups, but it is notable that only 2 weeks of treatment was applied, making it difficult to extrapolate these results to more modern applications of TMS therapy.

For the second study, 77 patients were randomized to receive either rTMS 5 days a week for 4 weeks (20 treatments) or treatment 3 days a week for 6 weeks (18 treatments) [15]. When assessed at 4 weeks, the patients who received daily treatment had improved to a greater degree. However, similar efficacy was achieved by the two groups when end of treatment assessments were compared. This indicated that more widely spaced treatment resulted in a slower response, but a response of a similar degree of efficacy.

6.3.2 More Intense Approaches

In contrast to this research, studies have also investigated more intensive treatment schedules. Highly intensive or accelerated treatment schedules are addressed in more detail in Chap. 10. A number of studies have however investigated the use of twice-daily rTMS, typically over half the duration that a standard daily course of rTMS would be applied. The study showed limited benefits of twice-daily treatment over sham but in a fairly small sample [16]. Significantly greater therapeutic effects were reported in a second study [17]. Of note, greater effects were seen with twice-rather once-daily rTMS and much greater than sham. However, the overall dose was not balanced between the twice- and once-daily groups so it was not clear whether the additional benefit of twice-daily treatment was not just an overall effect of dose and similar benefits would have been seen in the once-daily group if the treatment included the same dose over a longer period of time. In addition to these studies, two retrospective reports have presented analyses comparing once- to twice-daily responses and described faster but not greater therapeutic response with twice-daily treatment [18, 19]. A recent open-label analysis found greater responses to a twice-daily protocol in elderly versus younger patients without safety issues arising in the older group [20].

In a different approach, we have some very limited experience in the provision of treatment 7 days per week. The patients treated in this way mostly have not been noted to respond more quickly and on several occasions have actually required further treatment sessions such that the overall treatment duration remained approximately 4 weeks. On the basis of these initial findings, we did not progress to do a formal study of 7 days a week treatment.

Overall, the current evidence base does not support the routine use of twice-daily treatment in the absence of substantive sham-controlled or noninferiority trials.

6.3.3 Missing Sessions

Trials to date have varied considerably in how they have dealt with missed treatment sessions or extended session breaks, for example, over long weekends. In our experience, treatment can successfully proceed when patients have missed individual treatment sessions, but it would seem sensible to try and provide at least three treatment sessions within each week period and to limit protracted breaks.

6.3.4 Treatment Duration

In regard to the duration of rTMS treatment courses, these have varied across time from 1 week in initial studies to 6 weeks or longer in studies published in recent years. One method of analysis has suggested that better clinical responses have been seen in more recent clinical trials than earlier studies; it is possible that the increasing duration of treatment is a factor in this improvement [21]. There does appear to be a progressive improvement in mood across time during treatment implying that longer courses of treatment are likely to result in better clinical outcomes. For example, there was a clear reduction, week by week, in depression severity across a

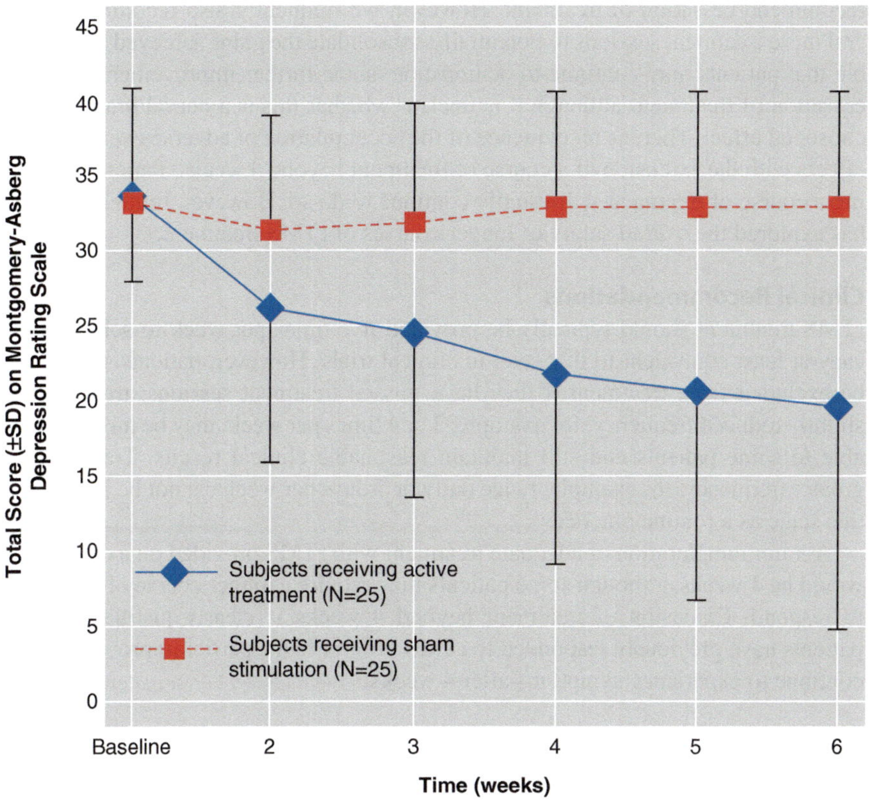

Fig. 6.1 The progressive reduction in depression scores in a clinical trial of bilateral rTMS seen in active treatment group over a 6-week period [6]

6-week period of time in the active treatment group in a trial of sequential bilateral rTMS conducted by our group (see Fig. 6.1) [6].

It is not clear, however, whether there is an optimal period of treatment. In a series of open-label clinical trials we have conducted, substantial response and remission rates have been achieved with 4 weeks of treatment. However, a subpopulation of patients does require a longer period of treatment to achieve substantial response. Although most patients will initially report some improvement during either week 2 or week 3 of treatment, occasionally patients do not experience mood shifts until considerably later. Four weeks seems to be a reasonably balanced minimal duration of adequate treatment although some recent research suggests that response may be predictable before this time point [22]. Whether to continue beyond 4 weeks of treatment in a patient who is not responding is a decision that should consider multiple factors: see further discussion in Chap. 7.

It can also be unclear when to cease treatment when a patient has responded clinically. Generally, patients should continue treatment while they are improving, but once clinical response has reached a plateau at an adequate level, we typically recommend cessation of treatment. However, we frequently also recommend several more treatment sessions to potentially consolidate the gains achieved. It is notable that patients may continue to demonstrate some further improvement after the cessation of treatment, although it is unclear whether this is a neural/brain or psychosocial effect. There is no evidence of the accumulation of adverse events or side effects with the extension of a course of treatment beyond 4 weeks. Patients tolerating a course of treatment will usually continue to do so. However, limited research has explored the overall safety of longer courses of rTMS treatment.

Clinical Recommendations

rTMS treatment should typically be provided five times per week to achieve efficacy at least equivalent to that seen in clinical trials. However, patients should not be excluded from treatment if they have missed treatment sessions: treatment at slightly reduced frequency, for example, 3 or 4 times per week, may be more acceptable to some patients and still maintain reasonable clinical results. Treatment at greater frequency, for example, twice daily or 7 days per week cannot be justified at this stage as a routine practice.

A minimum duration of adequate treatment with rTMS provided on a daily basis would be 4 weeks, although some patients may require a longer course of treatment to respond. Extension of treatment beyond 4 weeks is clearly justifiable when patients have previously responded to rTMS or have had a partial improvement but continue to experience symptoms after 4 weeks.

6.4 Concurrent Treatments

There are two potential issues with the consideration of concurrent medication treatment: whether there is a possibility of an impact on treatment efficacy, either favorable or not, and whether concurrent medication treatment increases the risk of adverse events such as seizure induction.

6.4.1 Potential Moderation of Efficacy

In regard to efficacy, a large number of clinical trials of rTMS in depression have included patients receiving antidepressant and often other forms of psychotropic medication. Several of the larger multisite trials (e.g., [23]), however, have been conducted in medication-free patients. When patients on medication have been enrolled in trials, it has been common to include only those who have failed to adequately respond to medication and where the dose of medication has been unchanged for a significant period of time prior to rTMS treatment, often 4 weeks. From the results of these trials, it appears that rTMS is effective in both medication-free and concurrently medicated patients. In fact, in a larger study published exploring this relationship, no difference in response was seen in patients taking antipsychotic medications but higher rates of response were seen in patients taking antidepressants (47.8% vs. 36.6%) or mood stabilizers (52.7% vs. 43.8%) compared to those that were not [24]. A recent meta-analysis also suggested that while rTMS was an effective treatment regardless, it was more effective in patients taking antidepressant medications compared to those who are not [25].

The situation is not as clear, however, when we consider the concurrent *commencement* of medication and rTMS treatment. Trials investigating this approach have generally found little difference between active and sham treatment, perhaps because the possible effects are more limited when concurrent treatment is commenced (e.g., [26]). Concurrently commencing treatment also raises a simple practical clinical issue: if a patient responds under these circumstances, it is not possible to know whether it was the medication, rTMS, or the combination, which resulted in clinical improvement. This uncertainty is likely to have implications for future recommendations regarding treatment options if the patient experiences a relapse.

One trial in another disorder did suggest that medication could potentially undermine rTMS response. This early study of the effect of rTMS treatment for auditory hallucinations in patients with schizophrenia found that patients responded more poorly when receiving rTMS concurrent with a mood stabilizer [27]. However, this has not been replicated in other hallucination studies, and analyses in substantial depression samples have not found this effect. In fact, analyses in depression samples have not found a moderating effect of any of the medication classes investigated.

A new issue in this domain has emerged in recent years following the publication of several reports that concurrent treatment with benzodiazepines may be associated with a more limited treatment response. The first of these found that benzodiazepine use was associated with a slightly reduced likelihood of improvement in 181 patients who had received a 6-week course of rTMS [28]. Benzodiazepine use was associated with less overall improvement and less improvement at week 2 of treatment. The second study involved the analysis of patterns of response to TMS and TBS. Patients receiving benzodiazepines had a lower likelihood of being in the so-called rapid response group, and there was statistically almost a relationship between benzodiazepine use and nonresponse (odds ratio = 2.25, CI = 0.99 and 5.11) [29]. We were not able to replicate this finding in a group of 185 patients treated across several trials [30]; an association between benzodiazepine use and overall depression improvement was found by Caulfield et al. [31] but another recent study recently found a lower rate of response in patients taking lorazepam than those who are not [32].

How should we interpret these rather conflicting results? First, it is important to note that all of these studies have been retrospective analyses. It is certainly possible that patients taking benzodiazepines have other clinical qualities that are associated with poor outcome and that it is not the use of these medications that directly is impacting treatment efficacy. However, until we have prospective meaningful data informing this question, it would be reasonable to advise patients to minimize the use of benzodiazepines during a course of treatment to mitigate any risk of poor outcomes.

6.4.2 Safety Considerations

In regard to safety considerations, the main concern is that concurrent medications may alter cortical excitability and contribute to a greater risk of seizure induction (Table 6.1). However, if medication is present at the time of the measurement of the RMT and the dose does not change over time, the effect on cortical excitability is likely to be at least partially controlled for in this initial measurement. However, changes in medication dose during treatment may result in an uncontrolled alteration of excitability increasing risk. Therefore, if substantial changes in medication doses are made, RMT levels should be re-measured and the prescribed rTMS intensity adjusted accordingly.

Of note, the greatest concerns in regard to safety of medication during rTMS treatment are likely to arise with medications known to predispose to seizures or alter excitability. Caution is warranted with clozapine, bupropion, tricyclic antidepressants, and stimulants such as amphetamine derivatives. However, a number of studies have included clozapine-treated patients in trials without complication, and we have treated depressed patients concurrently taking medication from all antidepressant classes. We have also treated without incident a number of patients receiving stimulants such as dexamphetamine. However, given the short duration of action of many of the medications in this class, we will often treat at a time of trough plasma levels. We also typically ensure that the measurement of the RMT and the provision of treatment occur at approximately the same time following medication dosing, for example, between 4 and 5 h after the morning or most recent dose.

Clinical Recommendations

There do not appear to be any adverse implications for the commencement of rTMS treatment in patients who are receiving a stable dose of antidepressant, mood stabilizing, or antipsychotic medications. Patients who have experienced a partial response to medication should not be weaned off this medication to undergo rTMS treatment unless for other specific reasons. There is no sensible rationale for the concurrent commencement of rTMS treatment and antidepressant medication and this should be avoided. Careful monitoring of the RMT and adjustment of treatment dose is required if medication is altered during treatment, especially when patients are receiving medications known to effect cortical excitability or the RMT. Until substantial prospective data is available, it would be prudent to advise patients to minimize the use of benzodiazepines in case this does impact on efficacy. However, caution should be taken to ensure that patients are not receiving rTMS treatment during a state of benzodiazepine withdrawal where there would be a significantly greater risk of seizure induction.

Table 6.1 Seizure risk associated with psychotropic medications

	Drug class	Drug name	Risk	Notes
Antidepressants	Tricyclic antidepressants (TCA)	Imipramine Amitriptyline Desipramine Nortriptyline Dothiepin	Majority of TCA medications pose low risk at therapeutic doses	Risk may be higher in genetic slow metabolizers, significantly increased risk at high dose/in overdose
		Clomipramine	Higher risk	
	Tetracyclic antidepressants	Maprotiline Amoxapine	Higher risk	
	Selective serotonin reuptake inhibitors (SSRIs)	All in class	Low risk	SSRIs can produce hyponatremia which can precipitate seizures
	Bupropion		Risk appears low to moderate in divided doses that total <400 mg/day and in slow release form	
	Phenylpiperazines	Trazodone Nefazodone	Low risk	
	Selective serotonin and norepinephrine reuptake inhibitors (SNRIs)	Venlafaxine	Low risk	Possibly higher risk at higher doses
	Mirtazapine		Low risk	
	Monoamine oxidase inhibitors (irreversible)	Phenelzine Tranylcypromine	Low risk	
	Monoamine oxidase inhibitors (reversible)	Moclobemide	Low risk	
	Noradrenaline reuptake inhibitors (NRIs)	Reboxetine	Low risk	
Antipsychotics	Phenothiazines	Chlorpromazine	Higher risk	
	High-potency typical antipsychotics	Haloperidol	Low risk	
	Atypical antipsychotics	Clozapine	Higher risk	Risk is significantly dose dependent

(continued)

Table 6.1 (continued)

	Drug class	Drug name	Risk	Notes
		Olanzapine	Possibly higher risk	
		Quetiapine	Possibly higher risk	
		Risperidone	Low risk	
		Ziprasidone	Low risk	
Mood stabilizers		Lithium	Possibly higher risk	Risk substantially increased at toxic plasma levels
Benzodiazepines		All in class	Low risk	High risk in withdrawal

Data partially summarized from review in [33]

References

1. George MS et al (2010) Daily left prefrontal transcranial magnetic stimulation therapy for major depressive disorder: a sham-controlled randomized trial. Arch Gen Psychiatry 67(5):507–516
2. O'Reardon J et al (2007) Efficacy and safety of transcranial magnetic stimulation in the acute treatment of major depression: a multi-site randomized controlled trial. Biol Psychiatry 62(11):1208–1216
3. Fitzgerald PB et al (2020) A pragmatic randomized controlled trial exploring the relationship between pulse number and response to repetitive transcranial magnetic stimulation treatment in depression. Brain Stimul 13(1):145–152
4. Carpenter L et al (2021) Comparison of clinical outcomes with two transcranial magnetic stimulation treatment protocols for major depressive disorder. Brain Stimul 14(1):173–180
5. Chen J et al (2013) Left versus right repetitive transcranial magnetic stimulation in treating major depression: a meta-analysis of randomised controlled trials. Psychiatry Res 210(3):1260–1264
6. Fitzgerald PB et al (2006) A randomized, controlled trial of sequential bilateral repetitive transcranial magnetic stimulation for treatment-resistant depression. Am J Psychiatry 163(1):88–94
7. Blumberger DM et al (2012) A randomized double-blind sham-controlled comparison of unilateral and bilateral repetitive transcranial magnetic stimulation for treatment-resistant major depression. World J Biol Psychiatry 13(6):423–435
8. Fitzgerald PB et al (2011) A randomized trial of unilateral and bilateral prefrontal cortex transcranial magnetic stimulation in treatment-resistant major depression. Psychol Med 41(6):1187–1196
9. Fitzgerald PB et al (2012) A double blind randomized trial of unilateral left and bilateral prefrontal cortex transcranial magnetic stimulation in treatment resistant major depression. J Affect Disord 139(2):193–198
10. Fitzgerald PB et al (2013) Equivalent beneficial effects of unilateral and bilateral prefrontal cortex transcranial magnetic stimulation in a large randomized trial in treatment-resistant major depression. Int J Neuropsychopharmacol 16(9):1975–1984
11. Berlim MT, Van den Eynde F, Daskalakis ZJ (2013) A systematic review and meta-analysis on the efficacy and acceptability of bilateral repetitive transcranial magnetic stimulation (rTMS) for treating major depression. Psychol Med 43(11):2245–2254

12. Chen JJ et al (2014) Bilateral vs. unilateral repetitive transcranial magnetic stimulation in treating major depression: a meta-analysis of randomized controlled trials. Psychiatry Res 219(1):51–57
13. Weissman CR et al (2018) Bilateral repetitive transcranial magnetic stimulation decreases suicidal ideation in depression. J Clin Psychiatry 79(3):17m11692
14. Turnier-Shea Y, Bruno R, Pridmore S (2006) Daily and spaced treatment with transcranial magnetic stimulation in major depression: a pilot study. Aust N Z J Psychiatry 40(9):759–763
15. Galletly C et al (2012) A randomized trial comparing repetitive transcranial magnetic stimulation given 3 days/week and 5 days/week for the treatment of major depression: is efficacy related to the duration of treatment or the number of treatments? Psychol Med 42(5):981–988
16. Loo CK et al (2007) A sham-controlled trial of the efficacy and safety of twice-daily rTMS in major depression. Psychol Med 37(3):341–349
17. Theleritis C et al (2017) Two versus one high-frequency repetitive transcranial magnetic stimulation session per day for treatment-resistant depression: a randomized sham-controlled trial. J ECT 33(3):190–197
18. Modirrousta M, Meek BP, Wikstrom SL (2018) Efficacy of twice-daily vs once-daily sessions of repetitive transcranial magnetic stimulation in the treatment of major depressive disorder: a retrospective study. Neuropsychiatr Dis Treat 14:309–316
19. Schulze L et al (2018) Number of pulses or number of sessions? An open-label study of trajectories of improvement for once-vs. twice-daily dorsomedial prefrontal rTMS in major depression. Brain Stimul 11(2):327–336
20. Desbeaumes Jodoin V, Miron JP, Lesperance P (2019) Safety and efficacy of accelerated repetitive transcranial magnetic stimulation protocol in elderly depressed unipolar and bipolar patients. Am J Geriatr Psychiatry 27(5):548–558
21. Gross M et al (2007) Has repetitive transcranial magnetic stimulation (rTMS) treatment for depression improved? A systematic review and meta-analysis comparing the recent vs. the earlier rTMS studies. Acta Psychiatr Scand 116(3):165–173
22. Lee JC, Wilson AC, Corlier J, Tadayonnejad R, Marder KG, Pleman CM, et al (2020) Strategies for augmentation of high-frequency left-sided repetitive transcranial magnetic stimulation treatment of major depressive disorder. J Affect Disord 277:964–969
23. O'Reardon JP et al (2007) Efficacy and safety of transcranial magnetic stimulation in the acute treatment of major depression: a multisite randomized controlled trial. Biol Psychiatry 62(11):1208–1216
24. Fitzgerald PB, Hoy KE, Anderson RJ, Daskalakis ZJ (2016) A study of the pattern of response to rtms treatment in depression. Depress Anxiety 33(8):746–53
25. Sehatzadeh S, Daskalakis ZJ, Yap B, Tu HA, Palimaka S, Bowen JM, et al (2019) Unilateral and bilateral repetitive transcranial magnetic stimulation for treatment-resistant depression: a meta-analysis of randomized controlled trials over 2 decades. J Psychiatry Neurosci 44(3):151–163
26. Herwig U et al (2007) Antidepressant effects of augmentative transcranial magnetic stimulation: randomised multicentre trial. Br J Psychiatry 191:441–448
27. Hoffman RE et al (2003) Transcranial magnetic stimulation of left temporoparietal cortex and medication-resistant auditory hallucinations. Arch Gen Psychiatry 60(1):49–56
28. Hunter AM, Minzenberg MJ, Cook IA, Krantz DE, Levitt JG, Rotstein NM, et al (2019) Concomitant medication use and clinical outcome of repetitive Transcranial Magnetic Stimulation (rTMS) treatment of Major Depressive Disorder. Brain Behav 9(5):e01275
29. Kaster TS, Downar J, Vila Rodriguez F, Thorpe KE, Feffer K, Noda Y, et al (2019) Trajectories of Response to Dorsolateral Prefrontal rTMS in Major Depression: A THREE-D Study. Am J Psychiatry 176(5):367–375
30. Fitzgerald PB, Hoy KE, Daskalakis ZJ (2020) Left handedness and response to repetitive transcranial magnetic stimulation in major depressive disorder. World J Biol Psychiatry 1–5
31. Caulfield KA, Stern AP (2020) Therapeutic High-Frequency Repetitive Transcranial Magnetic Stimulation Concurrently Improves Mood and Anxiety in Patients Using Benzodiazepines. Neuromodulation 23(3):380–383

32. Deppe M, Abdelnaim M, Hebel T, Kreuzer PM, Poeppl TB, Langguth B, et al (2021) Concomitant lorazepam use and antidepressive efficacy of repetitive transcranial magnetic stimulation in a naturalistic setting. Eur Arch Psychiatry Clin Neurosci 271(1):61–67
33. Lee KC, Finley PR, Alldredge BK (2003) Risk of seizures associated with psychotropic medications: emphasis on new drugs and new findings. Expert Opin Drug Saf 2(3):233–247

Switching, Continuing, or Ending Treatment

7

Abstract

There are multiple time points at which a decision may need to be made in regard to how to progress with, switch, or end an rTMS protocol. In patients who are improving with treatment, 6 weeks followed by taper is a standard evidence-based approach to therapy. However, it is less clear when to stop treatment in a patient who is showing no clinical response whatsoever, and it may be reasonable to do this earlier, for example, after 4 weeks of treatment, in patients where there are other substantive treatment options to try. When stopping high-frequency left-sided treatment, switching to an alternative form of rTMS may be a sensible treatment option. The switch might involve the use of sequential bilateral rTMS (perhaps more commonly in a patient who is a partial responder), low-frequency right-sided rTMS, or a number of novel paradigms. Finally, the use of a measurement-based care algorithm to structure decision-making around rTMS therapy provision is an emerging approach that is likely to improve standardization of care and clinical outcomes.

7.1 Introduction

There are several related, important, and common clinical questions that we wish to address in this chapter. These have to do with the decisions that need to be made once a patient has commenced a course of rTMS therapy in regard to how long the treatment should continue for and whether it should be altered in any meaningful way, especially in the context of patients who are not responding adequately to their initial stimulation conditions. As is the case in most areas of therapeutics, clinical trials predominantly address the first step of clinical decision-making: should I treat a patient with X or Y? The quality of research that addresses common garden clinical questions such as those that we will tackle in this chapter is often quite sparse

P. B. Fitzgerald, Z. J. Daskalakis, *rTMS Treatment for Depression*,
https://doi.org/10.1007/978-3-030-91519-3_7

and, as such, much more challenging to interpret. Therefore, practice tends to evolve much more variably and in a manner that depends on individual experiences and opinions.

There is, beyond the evolution of individual and somewhat idiosyncratic clinical practice, one other alternative, which is the development of algorithms for measurement-based care (MBC). MBC is based on the concept that decision-making for patients undergoing treatment should be informed by concrete measurements of clinical progress. In other words, patients undergoing rTMS would be receiving structured clinical evaluations usually using a depression rating scale at specific time intervals. Decisions on continuation, ceasing, or potentially switching treatment would be made based upon the progress of treatment as assessed on these measures. As an extension, rTMS therapy might be included in a broader treatment algorithm that is structured within the MBC framework. At this stage we are only just beginning to see the emergence of MBC protocols informing the use of rTMS, for example [1], but we suspect that this will play a greater role in the structure of treatment provision with interventional therapy such as rTMS going forward.

7.2 How Long Is Long Enough?

7.2.1 Patients Showing Improvement

The first aspect of this question is how long should one continue a course of TMS treatment for. This is relatively straightforward in the case of somebody who is having a substantial clinical response. Clinical trials have demonstrated that a longer course of treatment results in a continued improvement in depressive symptoms, and achieving the greatest degree of improvement possible is clearly desirable in both the short term and long term. Beyond patients just getting better, it seems likely that the degree of benefit achieved is likely to predict how long somebody is likely to stay well following the end of a course of TMS. In other words, somebody who has gone into complete remission is more likely to experience a sustained benefit than somebody who has only had a partial amelioration of the symptoms.

In this context, continuing to a full 6 weeks of treatment and then undertaking a taper over an additional 2 weeks, the protocol utilized in the pivotal Neuronetics trial would be a highly suitable option for most patients achieving a good clinical outcome. The describing pattern of clinical response in multiple randomized studies tends to show a progression of clinical improvement that continues right up until the end of treatment, no matter how long the treatment trial goes for. In fact, in many studies clinical response does not appear to a plateaued at the end of the conduct of the clinical trial. A good example of this was our first study of sequential bilateral treatment, one of the first studies that extended treatment to 6 weeks. We saw a significant improvement week to week throughout the 6 weeks of the study but this had not obviously plateaued at the end [2]. In a study which investigated the effects of further periods of treatment in patients included in the George et al. large multisite trial published in 2010 [3], this additional treatment was associated with improved remission rates [4]. These were patients who had shown a partial improvement with initial TMS treatment, and perhaps not surprisingly they continue to improve when the treatment duration was extended. In a similar manner, ongoing lower intensity treatment (twice weekly) with deep TMS following an initial treatment trial was associated with a progressive increase across time in response rates (an overall 8% increase) [5].

Therefore, certainly in somebody who is improving, longer does seem better and it would seem reasonable that this may ideally involve an extension beyond 6 weeks in a smaller subset of patients. In the consensus guidelines developed by the clinical TMS society [6], it was described that members of the society would occasionally extend treatment beyond 6 weeks in patients considered to be partial responders, especially those continuing to improve. However, extending treatment beyond 6 weeks should be something that should only occur after a very clear discussion and provision of informed consent given the lack of evidence supporting longer treatment durations.

In contrast, it is certainly possible that patients will have a marked improvement before the end of 6 weeks and they may well come a point where it is sensible to transition to a taper more rapidly. For example, if somebody is in remission by the 4-week/20 treatment time points, continuing with daily treatment for another 2 weeks prior to tapering would seem to be unnecessary: it will certainly be demanding in terms of time and cost with questionable benefit.

7.2.2 Clinical Recommendations

Six weeks plus a potential period of tapering seems reasonable as a standard course of rTMS treatment in the majority of patients. In patients who are showing improvement, continuing for this full length of time would seem to be the most sensible option to achieve maximal clinical benefit. However, there will be certain circumstances where it will be reasonable to finish treatment sooner when patients have achieved a complete remission of depressive symptoms.

7.2.3 Nonresponders

At this stage, there is limited data on which to base definitive recommendations in regard to the management of patients who are failing to respond to a course of rTMS, especially when there is no improvement in symptoms whatsoever. As such, there is variation in practice in this regard. Most commonly, as illustrated in the consensus guidelines of members of the Clinical TMS Society [6], practice tends to involve ceasing treatment in nonresponders after between 4 and 6 weeks of therapy. Many clinicians would regard 4 weeks as a reasonable duration of treatment to establish whether patients are going to respond or not, and cease after this time, while others would continue for a full course of 6 weeks of treatments in most patients.

Whether one ceases earlier, or continues for a full 6 weeks of treatment, is likely to be at least in part influenced by the likely availability or efficacy of other treatment alternatives and other factors such as the acuity of the depression and ease of accessibility of treatment to patients. Undertaking a full 6 weeks of treatment in somebody who is not responding, holding out in case a patient may be a late responder, is more likely to be an attractive option in a patient who has had a greater range of other treatments and has fewer other options which are likely to have therapeutic benefit. One may well be much more inclined to stop earlier in a patient who is experiencing significant suicidal ideation and ECT has been considered as a viable alternative.

Beyond stopping treatment itself, this decision may also consider the possibility of altering the rTMS stimulation parameters, rather than continuing for a full 6 weeks of the initial treatment, which would have most likely been high-frequency left-sided rTMS. There is the possibility of switching to a second form of rTMS, either following the completion of a full course of treatment or at some interim time point. As has been discussed previously in Chap. 4, there are multiple forms of rTMS that have been demonstrated to be effective that could be offered as an alternative in patients who are failing to improve with standard left-sided treatment.

Unfortunately, only limited research has explored the potential benefits of switching treatment. The first of these studies switched a small number of nonresponders to either high-frequency left-sided TMS or low-frequency right-sided TMS to the alternative [7]. Three patients who switched from right-sided to left-sided treatment (out of 10) achieved treatment response and 0/7 patients who switched in the opposite direction but treatment was applied for only 2 weeks and at quite low dose. A second study investigated switching following a failed course of low-frequency right-sided stimulation with rTMS applied at 5 or 10 Hz to the left DLPFC [8]. A significant antidepressant effect was seen with no difference between 5 and 10 Hz stimulation but the response rate overall was again relatively low.

Several more recent studies are more directly relevant to considering switching from an initial course of left-sided treatment. In the first of these, 17 nonresponders switched from 10 Hz left rTMS to sequential bilateral treatment [9]. Four patients became responders following bilateral treatment. In a second study, McDonald et al. provided 4 weeks of low-frequency right-sided rTMS to patients who had failed to respond to a substantive course of high-frequency left-sided rTMS. Twenty-one of 81 patients (26%) responded to this course of right-sided stimulation [4]. In a third study, nonresponders to 3 weeks of high-frequency left-sided rTMS were randomized to continue with the same treatment for another 3 weeks or to switch and have 3 weeks of either low-frequency right or sequential bilateral rTMS [10]. Modest antidepressant effects were seen in all three groups with no significant differences seen between the three options. However, the study really did not have sufficient power to detect meaningful between-group differences in response rates post-switching. Finally, in a completely different approach, Feffer et al. found a 36% response rate when providing 1 Hz stimulation to the right orbitofrontal cortex in nonresponders to dorsomedial stimulation [11].

These studies suggest that there is a modest but nonsignificant chance that a patient switching to a different form of rTMS may well achieve benefits if not responding initially. It does, however, remain unclear whether the clinical benefits seen in the switching studies could have arisen just with continuing the original course of treatment longer: is this just an overall effect of dose of stimulation and time or is there something specific about responding to a different stimulation approach?

Clinical decision-making in this area is also slightly confounded by the clinical observation that some patients will have a significantly delayed response to a course of therapy. We have repeatedly seen over time the example of patients who have finished a course of rTMS, with limited or even no response, and then found their mood improve, sometimes quite dramatically, in the weeks after they finish treatment. Therefore, it can make sense to offer the patient a break from treatment, following the completion of an initial unsuccessful course, to see whether they do get a delayed response. If this doesn't occur, the second course of a different form of TMS can be offered at a somewhat later time point. Again, it is worth emphasizing that decision-making in this regard needs to consider the other treatment option available and the individual circumstances of the patient.

Deep TMS (dTMS) as an Alternative Treatment Option

The discussion in this chapter is focused almost universally on treatment choices using a standard TMS system with a figure-of-eight coil as this is likely to be the options available to many people in clinical practice. However, switching to the use of dTMS is increasingly an option as dTMS systems become more widely available. There is minimal evidence available currently on the likelihood of clinical response when switching from standard rTMS to dTMS, but the substantial difference in effects of these two treatments makes this a very sensible and justifiable alternative in nonresponding patients to standard rTMS if dTMS is available. For further discussion of the role of dTMS, see Chap. 9.

7.3 Novel Options

A number of novel approaches have emerged in recent years that may prove to be useful in the nonresponding patient. The intermittent theta-burst priming of left DLPFC (iTBS-P) approach involves the application of iTBS immediately prior to the application of standard high-frequency left-sided rTMS. The iTBS is applied in a relatively standard fashion with 2-s trains, an 8-s intertrain interval, and a stimulation intensity of 120% of the RMT. Based on an observation that this form of iTBS-based priming could produce a significantly greater reduction in a pain protocol, initial research has illustrated that it might produce significant antidepressant benefits in patients who are nonresponders to standard left-sided treatment potentially to a greater degree than switching to sequential bilateral rTMS [1].

An alternative approach would be to apply treatment to a completely novel stimulation target. In this regard, one possibility is the dorsomedial area of the prefrontal cortex (DMPFC). There is reasonable emerging data from non-sham-controlled studies that antidepressant effects may arise from stimulation of the DMPFC with those seen with both standard 10 Hz rTMS and iTBS approaches in a large comparative trial [12]. Stimulation of the DMPFC does not produce significant cognitive side effects when stimulated alone or in combination with activation of the DLPFC [13, 14]. However, no sham-controlled data of stimulation at this site has yet been published.

There is also preliminary evidence for a second prefrontal stimulation site, in this case the right lateral orbitofrontal cortex (OFC). Stimulation of this site in 42 patients (a mixture of medication and DMPFC rTMS nonresponsive patients) demonstrated that 1 Hz stimulation was safe and produced a response rate of 37% [11].

7.3.1 Clinical Recommendations

Options for the treatment of nonresponding patients are presented in Fig. 7.1 and Box 7.1. In general, continuation of the current form of treatment makes the most sense in patients who are showing any degree of significant and ongoing improvement. Switching to sequential bilateral treatment should be considered in patients who have improved but only to a limited degree or where improvement has stalled. Patients who have failed to show any improvement after 20 or 30 high-frequency left-sided TMS sessions can potentially be offered a trial of low-frequency right-sided stimulation or a novel treatment paradigm such as bilateral TBS, iTBS-P, or stimulation of a novel target such as the dorsal medial prefrontal cortex.

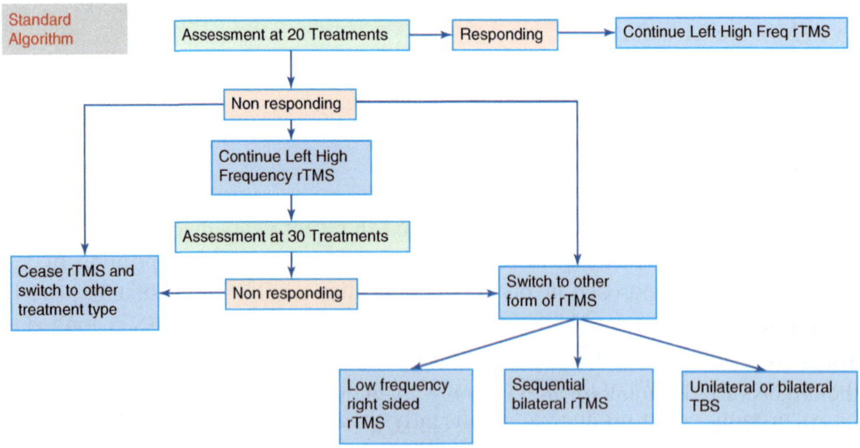

Fig. 7.1 Options in the treatment of the nonresponding patient

7.4 Clinical Decision-Making and the Measurement-Based Care Approach

An alternative method for the structuring of decision-making during rTMS therapy is the use of a measurement-based care (MBC) algorithm. MBC involves the use of a measurement, or multiple measurements, of symptom severity to help inform and determine specific treatment decisions. MBC has been demonstrated to improve overall quality of care and enhance clinical outcomes for patients in different aspects of psychiatric practice. In addition, patients engaged in MBC protocols tend to remain in treatment for longer. There is now emerging evidence that MBC protocols can be effectively integrated outside of research protocols into standard psychiatric clinical care.

Box 7.1 Treatment Alternatives at Interim Assessment (Most Commonly After 20 Treatments)

In remission: In patients who have already achieved clear remission after 20 treatments, transition to a tapering of acute treatment is a reasonable consideration.

Responding: Patients who are clearly significantly improving in response to a course of treatment after 20 sessions should continue treatment to the 30-session time point to try and achieve full remission of symptoms.

Partial response: In the circumstances where there has been only very limited response after 20 sessions or an initial response has "stalled," consider a switch to sequential bilateral rTMS. This will allow the patient to continue receiving the intervention that has provided some benefit to date but to also access a different treatment modality.

Nonresponse: In the circumstances of clear nonresponse after 20 treatments, there are several reasonable treatment options (see Fig. 7.1) that are worthy of consideration and discussion with the patient. A decision should be made in collaboration with the treatment following a discussion of these treatment options. Deep TMS should be considered if available.

Given the multiple potential decision points that can occur during a course of rTMS therapy, MBC approaches could be used to guide the choice of treatment options: providing structure, consistency of care, and decision-making. To date there has been minimal research on the implementation of MBC models in clinical care. Some preliminary reports are emerging describing outcomes of patients treated with instruction algorithms such as that by Lee et al. [1]. In that study, all patients commencing rTMS therapy for depression were treated with high-frequency left-sided rTMS. Patients were assessed with the inventory of depressive symptoms (self-rated) (IDS-SR) rating scale at baseline and after every five treatments. Treatment could be modified after every five treatments in patients not achieving a greater than 20% improvement in their IDS-SR score. Modification initially

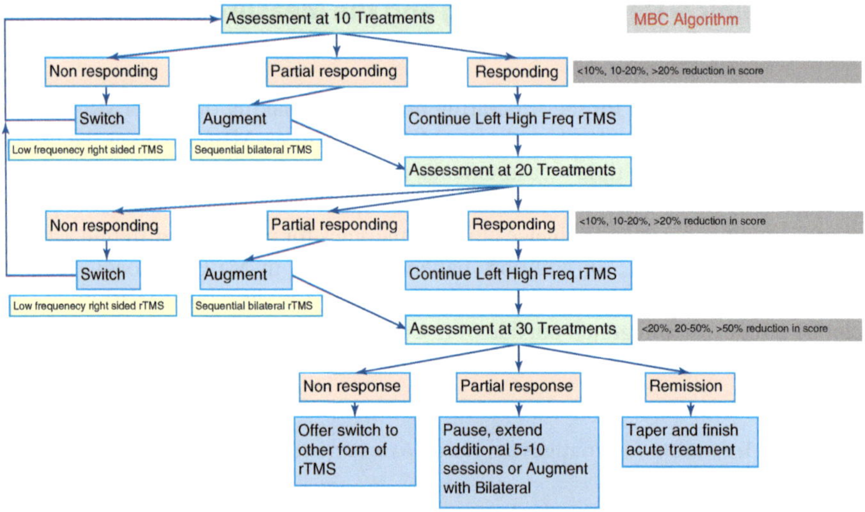

Fig. 7.2 A potential measurement-based care treatment algorithm

included a switch to sequential bilateral treatment but later in the study involved the addition of an intermittent theta-burst priming protocol. Of note, the switching treatment was not mandatory: patients could continue with high-frequency left-sided treatment if their training condition judged that they were improving in a manner that might indicate that they might eventually "derive greater benefit." Although this is a relatively simple implementation of the MBC approach, it does demonstrate the use of a structured rating scale to directly inform treatment decision-making. A possible example of elements of an MBC algorithm is shown in Fig. 7.2.

References

1. Lee JC et al (2020) Strategies for augmentation of high-frequency left-sided repetitive transcranial magnetic stimulation treatment of major depressive disorder. J Affect Disord 277:964–969
2. Fitzgerald PB et al (2006) A randomized, controlled trial of sequential bilateral repetitive transcranial magnetic stimulation for treatment-resistant depression. Am J Psychiatry 163(1):88–94
3. George MS et al (2010) Daily left prefrontal transcranial magnetic stimulation therapy for major depressive disorder: a sham-controlled randomized trial. Arch Gen Psychiatry 67(5):507–516
4. McDonald WM et al (2011) Improving the antidepressant efficacy of transcranial magnetic stimulation: maximizing the number of stimulations and treatment location in treatment-resistant depression. Depress Anxiety 28(11):973–980
5. Yip AG et al (2017) 61% of unmedicated treatment resistant depression patients who did not respond to acute TMS treatment responded after four weeks of twice weekly deep TMS in the Brainsway pivotal trial. Brain Stimul 10(4):847–849
6. Perera T et al (2016) The clinical TMS Society consensus review and treatment recommendations for TMS therapy for major depressive disorder. Brain Stimul 9(3):336–346
7. Fitzgerald PB et al (2003) A double-blind placebo controlled trial of transcranial magnetic stimulation in the treatment of depression. Arch Gen Psychiatry 60:1002–1008

8. Fitzgerald PB et al (2009) A study of the effectiveness of high-frequency left prefrontal cortex transcranial magnetic stimulation in major depression in patients who have not responded to right-sided stimulation. Psychiatry Res 169(1):12–15
9. Cristancho P et al (2019) Crossover to bilateral repetitive transcranial magnetic stimulation: a potential strategy when patients are not responding to unilateral left-sided high-frequency repetitive transcranial magnetic stimulation. J ECT 35(1):3–5
10. Fitzgerald PB et al (2018) Exploring alternative rTMS strategies in non-responders to standard high frequency left-sided treatment: a switching study. J Affect Disord 232:79–82
11. Feffer K et al (2018) 1Hz rTMS of the right orbitofrontal cortex for major depression: safety, tolerability and clinical outcomes. Eur Neuropsychopharmacol 28(1):109–117
12. Bakker N et al (2015) rTMS of the dorsomedial prefrontal cortex for major depression: safety, tolerability, effectiveness, and outcome predictors for 10 Hz versus intermittent theta-burst stimulation. Brain Stimul 8(2):208–215
13. Kavanaugh BC et al (2018) Neurocognitive effects of repetitive transcranial magnetic stimulation with a 2-coil device in treatment-resistant major depressive disorder. J ECT 34(4):258–265
14. Schulze L et al (2016) Cognitive safety of dorsomedial prefrontal repetitive transcranial magnetic stimulation in major depression. Eur Neuropsychopharmacol 26(7):1213–1226

8 The Use of Deep Transcranial Magnetic Stimulation in Depression

Abstract

Deep TMS (dTMS) is a form of rTMS that involves the use of a specific TMS coil to produce stimulation to a greater depth of the cortex than is achieved with traditional coils such as the figure-of-eight coil. dTMS was initially developed using a number of Hesed or H-coils although coils including the double cone coil can be used to produce similar effects in some brain regions. dTMS coils typically produce magnetic field that penetrates further into the brain, but this is accompanied by significant stimulation of a broader area of the cortical surface. dTMS has been shown to have significant antidepressant effects and proof of clinical use and more recently to have therapeutic benefit in other applications including obsessive-compulsive disorder and smoking cessation.

8.1 Introduction

Deep TMS (dTMS) refers to the use of a TMS system to stimulate the brain in a manner that penetrates to a greater depth of penetration than is typically achieved with a standard TMS coil. The first description of a coil able to provide transcranial magnetic stimulation of deep brain regions was presented in the paper by Roth et al. (2002) and several years later in a paper reporting modeling of the electrical field distribution produced by these Hesed or H-coils [1, 2]. These studies showed that the H-coil was capable of providing stimulation and a significantly greater depth of penetration but with also a significantly greater degree of stimulation of the cortical surface. The effects in humans were first reported in a safety study of two differing H-coil designs published in 2007 [3]. Since that time, a number of different coil designs have been investigated and tested, often with electrical field modeling. Variations of the original H-coil have been developed for targeting different brain regions, and studies have shown that double cone coils can also produce significant

P. B. Fitzgerald, Z. J. Daskalakis, *rTMS Treatment for Depression*, https://doi.org/10.1007/978-3-030-91519-3_8

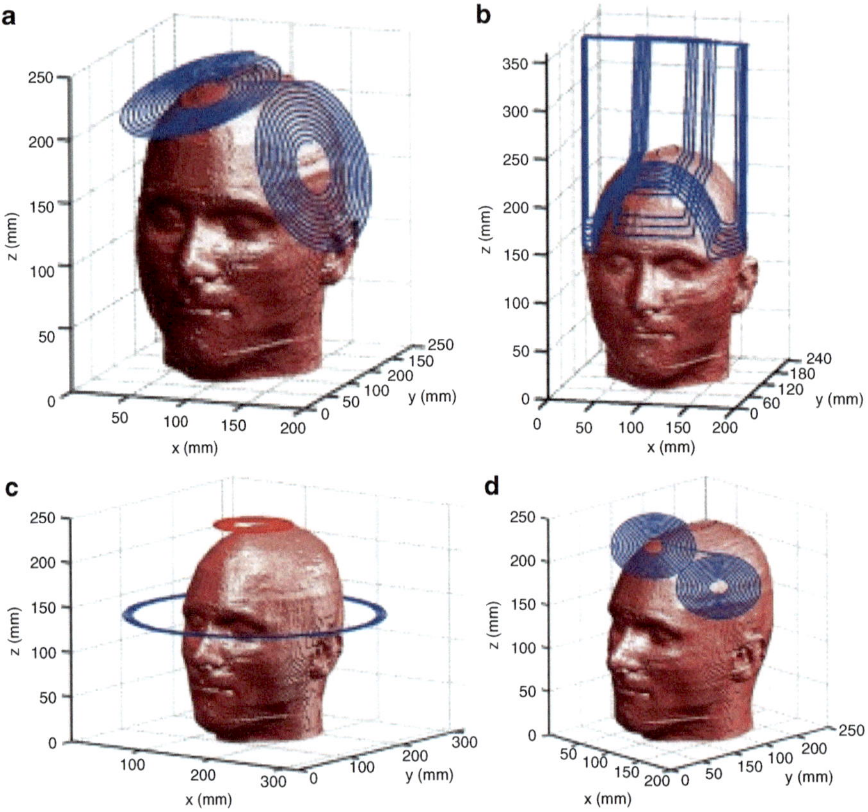

Fig. 8.1 Head model showing the configuration of (**a**) double cone, (**b**) H, (**c**) HCA, and (**d**) figure-of-eight coils. (From Lu M, Ueno S. Comparison of the induced fields using different coil configurations during deep transcranial magnetic stimulation. PLoS One. 2017;12(6):e0178422. Open access-permission not required for use)

deep stimulation although both of these type of coil systems produce wider superficial cortical stimulation and some coils come with a risk of optical nerve stimulation [4–6] (Fig. 8.1).

8.2 Clinical Application of dTMS

The main impetus for the development of clinical applications of dTMS has been the commercial activity of the company Brainsway Ltd. who have commercialized the application of a family of H-coils, now in an increasing range of clinical applications. The primary application of this technology has been the use of the H1 coil in the treatment of patients with major depressive disorder. Following an initial pilot study in 65 patients exploring different treatment parameters [7], the primary data establishing the efficacy of dTMS has come from a single large randomized controlled trial that was used to achieve device registration in the USA and elsewhere [8]. In this study, 212 patients with MDD received active or sham stimulation over 4 weeks on a daily basis and then biweekly for 12 weeks. Of note, efficacy data from the per-protocol (but not the intention to treat) analysis showed significant differences between active and sham stimulation with clinical benefits persistent across the maintenance phase. In addition, significant benefits were seen on a variety of secondary outcomes. The results of this trial were sufficient to lead to clinical approval in the USA and the progressive expansion of the availability of dTMS over recent years.

The effectiveness of dTMS has been evaluated in a number of other research trials. For example, short-term efficacy was demonstrated in a group of patients ($N = 50$) with depression in bipolar affective disorder [9]. A study has also shown antidepressant effects in patients with late-life depression [10].

There has also been one independently funded and quite substantial attempt to compare dTMS with standard rTMS. This trial involved the application of 20 sessions of either TMS treatment (or medication alone) in a randomized fashion to 228 patients with major depressive disorder. Both rTMS and rTMS produced superior antidepressant effects than medication alone, but there was no difference between the two forms of TMS on the primary outcome assessment. There were some benefits seen, however, in the dTMS group on some secondary outcome measures although the dTMS group also reported a higher rate of side effects.

It is worthy of note that typical applications of dTMS have used short bursts of 20 Hz stimulation rather than the 10 Hz which is typically used with standard high-frequency rTMS applied with a figure-of-eight coil. At this stage it is quite unclear whether there is a relationship between variation in frequency of this sort and clinical benefits.

Common Treatment Parameters for Deep TMS Using the Brainsway H-Coil*

- 18 Hz
- 2 s trains
- 20 s intertrain interval
- 55 trains
- 1980 pulses
- 120% of the RMT

*These were the stimulation parameters used in the pivotal dTMS approval trial.

8.3 Safety of dTMS

There was one seizure reported in the pivotal registration trial described above [8] and a seizure in the first patient enrolled in a trial in adolescent depression [11]. The manufacturer, Brainsway, following the main dTMS system, and the only dTMS systems using H-coils, has recently published a paper describing seizure rates utilizing data systematically collected from clinics using their TMS system between 2010 and October 2020. Over this time there were 55 seizures, of which only 14 occurred when the instructions for use of the deep TMS system were followed fully. Outside of this group of 14 patients, a number of seizures occurred when patients were treated without an RMT check following medication changes, when there had been incidences of substance use in 24 h prior to treatment or poor sleep the night before therapy. The overall seizure frequency was 6 per 10,000 patients and 2 per 10,000 patients where the protocol was fully followed. Of importance, no patients required intervention for the cessation of a seizure and no injuries or long-term complications accrued.

8.4 Not All Deep TMS Involves the Use of an H-Coil

Although the vast majority of treatment that is occurring clinically with TMS uses one or other of the H-coils produced by Brainsway, electric field modeling indicates that dTMS stimulation can be achieved with double cone coils and other forms of coil configuration that can be connected to standard TMS systems. The most widely available of these other coils able to produce deeper TMS penetration is the so-called double cone coil. A double cone coil is a larger figure-of-eight coil with a significant degree of angulation between the two wings of the coil [12]. A double cone coil produced by the device manufacturer MagVenture has been approved for the treatment of obsessive-compulsive disorder (OCD) following the initial approval of the Brainsway H7 coil in OCD, but no coil other than the Brainsway H1 coil has been approved for use in depression.

A third coil configuration which has been designed but not used significantly in clinical practice is the halo circular assembly (HCA) coil which involves a large circular coil placed around the head and a smaller coil placed on the cortical surface. Finally, preliminary data was collected in the early 2010s on the use of a two- [13] or four-coil array for the production of deep but focal TMS stimulation, but the commercial development of this system has not progressed since that time.

8.4.1 Expanding Applications of dTMS

As alluded to in the previous section, interest in the use of dTMS has expanded beyond application of these treatments in depression. The first FDA-approved indication for dTMS using the Brainsway system outside of depression was in the treatment of OCD. A Brainsway H-coil has also been approved for use in the treatment of smoking addiction/to aid in smoking cessation. A recent multisite clinical trial failed to demonstrate the therapeutic efficacy of dTMS in PTSD (https://www.brainsway.com/news_events/brainsway-reports-results-of-interim-analysis-of-h7-deep-transcranial-magnetic-stimulation-study-in-post-traumatic-stress-disorder/), and clinical trials are underway in a variety of other conditions.

8.5 Conclusion and Clinical Recommendations

There is sufficient evidence for the use of dTMS as a standalone treatment for patients with depression as an alternative to standard forms of rTMS using a figure-of-eight coil, and this is reflected in the increasing use of dTMS in clinical practice. Switching to dTMS may also be a sensible option in patients who are failing to respond to a course of "standard" rTMS therapy.

References

1. Roth Y, Amir A, Levkovitz Y, Zangen A (2007) Three-dimensional distribution of the electric field induced in the brain by transcranial magnetic stimulation using figure-8 and deep H-coils. J Clin Neurophysiol 24(1):31–38
2. Roth Y, Zangen A, Hallett M (2002) A coil design for transcranial magnetic stimulation of deep brain regions. J Clin Neurophysiol 19(4):361–370
3. Levkovitz Y, Roth Y, Harel EV, Braw Y, Sheer A, Zangen A (2007) A randomized controlled feasibility and safety study of deep transcranial magnetic stimulation. Clin Neurophysiol 118(12):2730–2744
4. Gomez-Tames J, Hamasaka A, Hirata A, Laakso I, Lu M, Ueno S (2020) Group-level analysis of induced electric field in deep brain regions by different TMS coils. Phys Med Biol 65(2):025007
5. Guadagnin V, Parazzini M, Fiocchi S, Liorni I, Ravazzani P (2016) Deep transcranial magnetic stimulation: modeling of different coil configurations. IEEE Trans Biomed Eng 63(7):1543–1550
6. Lu M, Ueno S (2017) Comparison of the induced fields using different coil configurations during deep transcranial magnetic stimulation. PLoS One 12(6):e0178422
7. Levkovitz Y, Harel EV, Roth Y, Braw Y, Most D, Katz LN et al (2009) Deep transcranial magnetic stimulation over the prefrontal cortex: evaluation of antidepressant and cognitive effects in depressive patients. Brain Stimul 2(4):188–200
8. Levkovitz Y, Isserles M, Padberg F, Lisanby SH, Bystritsky A, Xia G et al (2015) Efficacy and safety of deep transcranial magnetic stimulation for major depression: a prospective multicenter randomized controlled trial. World Psychiatry 14(1):64–73
9. Tavares DF, Myczkowski ML, Alberto RL, Valiengo L, Rios RM, Gordon P et al (2017) Treatment of bipolar depression with deep TMS: results from a double-blind, randomized, parallel group, sham-controlled clinical trial. Neuropsychopharmacology 42(13):2593–2601
10. Kaster TS, Daskalakis ZJ, Noda Y, Knyahnytska Y, Downar J, Rajji TK et al (2018) Efficacy, tolerability, and cognitive effects of deep transcranial magnetic stimulation for late-life depression: a prospective randomized controlled trial. Neuropsychopharmacology 43(11):2231–2238
11. Cullen KR, Jasberg S, Nelson B, Klimes-Dougan B, Lim KO, Croarkin PE (2016) Seizure induced by deep transcranial magnetic stimulation in an adolescent with depression. J Child Adolesc Psychopharmacol 26(7):637–641
12. Lontis ER, Voigt M, Struijk JJ (2006) Focality assessment in transcranial magnetic stimulation with double and cone coils. J Clin Neurophysiol 23(5):462–471
13. Carpenter LL, Aaronson ST, Clarke GN, Holtzheimer PE, Johnson CW, McDonald WM et al (2017) rTMS with a two-coil array: safety and efficacy for treatment resistant major depressive disorder. Brain Stimul 10(5):926–933

9 Theta-Burst Stimulation (TBS)

Abstract

Theta-burst stimulation (TBS) is a patterned form of rTMS which involves the application of short bursts (three pulses) applied at high frequency (most commonly 50 Hz) and repeated at theta frequency (typically 5 Hz). Physiological data indicates that TBS can produce similar effects to high- and low-frequency rTMS but with a much-reduced length of stimulation application. Considerable research is ongoing to define the best parameters for TBS application to maximize effects and efficiency. In the meantime, clinical trials have demonstrated that unilateral and bilateral forms of TBS can have antidepressant efficacy and intermittent TBS (iTBS) has been shown to have similar efficacy to standard left prefrontal rTMS in large noninferiority trials. This has led to FDA approval in the USA and increased clinical application. iTBS applied to the left DLPFC appears to be a significant clinical value although further research is required to optimize the use of TBS in general and to fully establish its role in clinical therapeutics.

9.1 Introduction

Theta-burst stimulation (TBS) is a form of patterned rTMS [1]. It typically involves the application of a very short (e.g., three pulses) high-frequency bursts: usually, but not always, at 50 Hz. These bursts are then repeated at theta frequency (usually 5 Hz). During continuous TBS (cTBS), stimulation is continued for 40 s in a single train. During intermittent TBS (iTBS), 2-s trains are repeated with 8-s intervals for a total time of typically 190 s [1]. In physiological experiments investigating the

P. B. Fitzgerald, Z. J. Daskalakis, *rTMS Treatment for Depression*,
https://doi.org/10.1007/978-3-030-91519-3_9

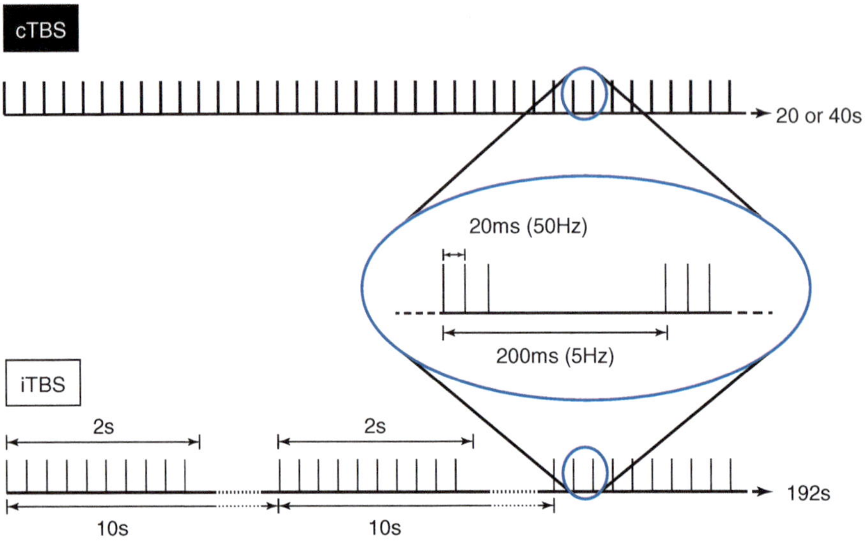

Fig. 9.1 An outline of the TBS pulse sequencing showing high-frequency (typically 50 Hz) three pulse bursts being repeated at theta frequency (typically 5 Hz) in both the intermittent and continuous TBS protocols. (Adapted from Chen et al. review paper, get permission)

application of these forms of TBS applied to the motor cortex, they have opposite effects with iTBS producing an increase, and cTBS a decrease, in cortical excitability. However, there is considerable individual variability in the direction and degree of these effects achieved in single session studies in healthy control subjects (Fig. 9.1).

Why Is It Called Theta-Burst Stimulation?

The designation theta-burst stimulation refers to the application of "bursts" of stimulation at theta frequency. These bursts of stimulation are actually the triplet pulses (three pulses together) typically applied at 50 Hz or gamma frequency.

The terminology theta or gamma frequency comes from the neuroscience literature describing the patterns of neuronal oscillations, specifically the frequency that clusters of nerve cells fire at, most typically recorded with electroencephalography (EEG). Oscillations in the 4–8 Hz range are typically referred to as theta oscillations and those in the 30–80 Hz range are regarded as gamma oscillations. Perhaps a better term for theta-burst stimulation would be theta-gamma stimulation.

9.2 TBS and Its Effects on Brain Function

The first human studies demonstrating the effects of TBS investigated its effects on the motor cortex. In the first of these studies, Huang et al. reported the effects of 5 or 15 rTMS pulses applied at 50 Hz and repeated at 5 Hz intervals. This study showed substantial and long-lasting effects on motor cortical excitability compared with single pulse TMS applied at the same intensity [2]. A subsequent study investigated the effects of the application of three pulses at 50 Hz, in much the same way that TBS is now done, repeated at 5 Hz for durations of 20–192 s. This study reported differential effects on motor cortical excitability determined by the pattern of TBS applied: cTBS applied three 50 Hz pulses at 5 Hz uninterrupted for 40 s and produced a reduction in motor evoked potential (MEP) amplitude, indicating reduced motor cortical excitability. Intermediate TBS (imTBS) applied three 50 Hz pulses at 5 Hz over 5 s, followed by 15 s of inactivity, with repeated cycles that continued for 110 seconds. This stimulation pattern induced no apparent conditioning response. iTBS also applied with three 50 Hz pulses at 5 Hz but over 2 s, followed by 8 s of rest, with repeated cycles that continued for 192 s. This iTBS stimulation pattern led to increased MEP amplitude, suggestive of increased motor cortical excitability. The direct effects of TBS paradigms on motor cortical excitability have been replicated in a number of studies although in some they have not been clearly seen and there has been considerable interindividual and intraindividual variability in these effects reported [3–6].

The striking feature of TBS is that the studies using TBS in the motor cortex have shown that it can produce changes in cortical excitability with much briefer stimulation periods than with traditional rTMS [7]. For example, the typical iTBS session is of 3-min duration and a typical cTBS session of 40-s duration. Physiological experiments in healthy control subjects suggest that lengthening the duration of TBS applied when using either paradigms does not tend to produce greater effects, and sometimes can reduce the changes in cortical excitability or even convert excitatory effects to inhibitory or vice versa [8, 9].

A limited range of studies have also explored similar effects of TBS outside of the motor cortex, in particular with prefrontal stimulation [10]. For example, we did not find that applying an iTBS train twice produced greater effects on cortical excitability than just applying the same paradigm once when assessing the effects of stimulation on prefrontal excitability using combined TMS-EEG methods [11].

There is also some uncertainty as to the optimal stimulation intensity to be used when applying TBS. The vast majority of physiological studies developing these paradigms actually applied TBS at quite low subthreshold stimulation intensities, usually the equivalent of about 70% of the RMT: clearly much lower than the stimulation intensities used in a standard rTMS therapeutic paradigms. When we evaluated the electrophysiological effects of iTBS applied at either 50%, 75%, or 100% of the RMT, we found that the greatest effects were produced with the intermediate stimulation intensity (75%) [12].

Some studies have also used neuroimaging methods to study the effects of TBS on brain activity. For example, using functional MRI, cTBS was found to suppress metabolic activity [13] and induce regionally specific patterns of activation and suppressed neural activity [14]. In a second study, iTBS applied to the motor cortex was shown to change local cerebral blood perfusion but also to have effects on distally network connected regions [15]. Brain effects of TBS have also been explored in the context of the treatment of depression. A randomized controlled trial investigating the effects of ten sessions of iTBS, cTBS, combined iTBS/cTBS, and sham stimulation included pre- and post-TBS positron emission tomography (PET) imaging. This showed that active stimulation induced significant metabolic changes in fronto-cingulo-temporal circuitry not seen with sham stimulation [16]. TBS-related perfusion changes have also been investigated with near-infrared spectroscopy (NIRS). TBS induced transient deoxygenation in regions both local and distal to the stimulation site(s), which was not seen with sham TBS [17, 18]. Although these preliminary findings suggest that TBS produces both local and distal changes in brain activity, how these changes differ from those induced with standard forms of rTMS and how they relate to clinical effects remain unclear.

9.3 TBS in Depression

9.3.1 Preliminary Clinical Trials

The first attempts to use TBS to treat patients with depression were reported in studies back in 2009 and 2010. Holzer and Padberg described an open-label series of seven patients who received daily ITBS to the left DLPFC with three patients achieving remission of depression after 3 weeks of treatment [19]. In the same year Christyakov et al. described the results of an open-label study where 33 patients received either left-sided iTBS or right-sided cTBS with the latter administered in three different dosage configurations. More than 55% of patients recorded a clinical response to treatment with high dose (longer cTBS trains) being reported as more effective [20].

Since these initial reports there have been a series of moderate sized sham-controlled randomized trials with sample sizes all below 100 (e.g., [21–26]). These have included iTBS to the left DLPFC, cTBS to the right, and sequential bilateral combination treatment in a variety of different protocols. The treatment protocols in these studies have also been quite variable in terms of stimulation intensities relative to the RMT (80–110%), course durations (10–30 sessions), and total pulses applied (18,000 to 72,000 pulses). For example, a recent study showed greater effects of a prolonged 1800 pulse iTBS protocol compared to sham stimulation (iTBS was not superior to a standard rTMS arm) [27].

A meta-analysis summarizing the results of the preliminary trials was published in 2017 including 5 reports with 221 patients [28]. This analysis concluded that TBS produced greater response rates than sham but there was not a significant difference in terms of remission. Dropout rates were actually numerically lower in the active than the sham groups, indicating a high degree of tolerability/acceptability.

9.3.2 TBS in Bipolar Depression

Of note, almost all of the trials to date have been for patients experiencing a major depressive episode except for one in patients with depression in the context of bipolar affective disorder [21]. However, the use of iTBS in bipolar depression has been followed up in a recent small randomized controlled trial comparing 4 weeks of daily iTBS to sham stimulation at 120% of the RMT [29]. The trial was terminated early after the randomization of 37 patients as a preliminary analysis showed no difference between the active and sham stimulation groups. Two episodes of hypomania were noted, one during double-blind treatment and one during an open-label treatment phase.

9.3.3 The Three-D Trial

The most substantive TBS trial conducted to date, and the one which has had the most influence on the field, is the so-called Three-D study published in 2018 [30]. This was a noninferiority trial: a noninferiority trial sets out to demonstrate that one treatment is not inferior to an existing effective treatment option. The study compared a single daily 600 pulse train of iTBS applied to the left DLPFC to a single daily course of 10 Hz rTMS (75 trains) applied to the same site total of 414 randomized subjects. There was no significant difference in outcomes after treatment. In fact, the difference between the two groups was 0.10 points on the Hamilton Rating Scale for depression, substantially under the predetermined cutoff of 2.25 points to indicate inferiority. Response rates for the rTMS and iTBS arms were 47% and 49%, while remission rates were 27% and 32%, respectively. Pain was rated as more intense in the iTBS group but dropout rates were lower across both groups and did not differ.

The results of this study have been considered a fairly definitive demonstration of the noninferiority of TBS when applied with a single 600 pulse train of iTBS to the left DLPFC. It is worth noting that iTBS in this study was applied at 120% of the RMT, and there is little information yet to suggest whether this is likely to be optimal or not. It is certainly a level at which TBS tends to be fairly uncomfortable in some patients as indicated by the higher rates of pain in this study report, but clearly treatment overall was tolerable and acceptable.

9.3.4 Other TBS Studies in Depression

Consistent with the use of rTMS in depression in general, almost all of the TBS studies have targeted the left DLPFC. However, a limited line of research has explored the application of TBS to the dorsomedial prefrontal cortex (DMPFC). In a large retrospective case series, 185 patients with treatment-resistant depression received 20–30 sessions of daily iTBS or 10 Hz rTMS applied to the DMPFC at

120% of the RMT. Comparable depression response and remission rates were reported between the two protocols [31].

Limited research has also started to explore the use of iTBS applied with a deep TMS H-configuration coil [32].

9.4 Use of Accelerated or Intensive Protocols

Due to the obvious efficiency with which TBS can be applied, it clearly lends itself to potential use in more intensive or accelerated protocols where higher doses of stimulation or multiple stimulation applications are applied each day, for a shorter period of time than a typical course of rTMS therapy. The aim behind this form of treatment approach can be to either achieve a more rapid clinical response, to try and achieve a greater clinical response due to the application of a higher stimulation dose, or to try and achieve clinical benefits more efficiently, requiring patients to attend clinical service on fewer occasions.

The first attempt to use TBS in some form of accelerated protocol involved a sham-controlled crossover study where 20 real or sham iTBS sessions were applied over 4 days before all participants were crossed over at the start of week 2 and the stimulation protocols repeated [23]. Statistically significant improvements in HDRS scores were observed across both study arms at the end of weeks 1 and 2 crossover design, making interpretation of the follow-up of the patient somewhat difficult.

We recently conducted a randomized blinded trial comparing an intensive application of iTBS applied to the left DLPFC to a standard course of 4 weeks of daily (5 days per week) 10 Hz rTMS [33]. Three iTBS treatments (600 pulses each) were given each day for 3 days in week 1, three treatments a day for 2 days in week 2, and three treatments in 1 day in week 3 and in week 4. Seventy-four patients received randomized treatment and we found no degree in mean reduction in depressive symptoms and the rate of remission or response between the two groups. No differences in side effect rates, adverse events, or cognitive performance were seen between the two groups.

Attention has been paid to the "SAINT" protocol developed at Stanford which is also an accelerated form of TBS stimulation. This involves the application of 50 iTBS sessions (1800 pulses per session, 50-min intersession interval) during 10 daily sessions over 5 consecutive days at 90% of the RMT and localized using functional connectivity and MRI-based neuronavigation. In an open-label series, this resulted in an impressive remission rate of 19 out of 21 patients but this requires replication in a controlled trial [34].

9.5 Safety of Theta-Burst Stimulation

The safety profile of TBS does not appear to be significantly different to that seen with standard rTMS therapy. TBS can induce the standard common side effects seen with TMS such as scalp discomfort or pain, facial jaw twitches, and headaches [35].

The risk of seizure induction with TBS stimulation is likely to be substantially related to stimulation intensity, as it is with other TMS paradigms although several seizures have been reported at modest stimulation intensities. For example, in one patient seizure was induced with cTBS applied at 80% of the RMT but to the right operculo-insular cortex (over the right Sylvian fissure) with an angled double cone coil designed for deep stimulation [36]. The second seizure was induced with cTBS applied to the left motor cortex at 100% of the RMT [37].

A systematic review evaluated the adverse events reported in 64 TBS studies, in a mixture of patients and healthy controls. One seizure was reported in greater than 4500 sessions of TBS [38]. The review concluded seizure risk with TBS is comparable with high-frequency rTMS protocols, where seizures have occurred in less than 0.1% of patients.

9.6 Practical Implementation

On the basis of the Three-D study, the use of iTBS was granted FDA approval in the USA in August 2018. More recently, the FDA also granted approval for the use of iTBS applied with the Brainsway deep TMS system based on a study of 146 patients who received treatment with either standard TMS or TBS through a deep TMS coil and which showed therapeutic equivalence (https://www.globenewswire.com/en/news-release/2021/04/26/2216716/17676/en/BrainsWay-Receives-FDA-Clearance-for-Three-Minute-Theta-Burst-Treatment-Protocol-for-Major-Depressive-Disorder.html#:~:text=(NASDAQ%20%26%20TASE%3A%20BWAY),minute%20protocol%20utilizing%20its%20proprietary). TBS protocols can be administered through equipment produced by most TMS manufacturers, and clearly the shorter duration of treatment makes this a potentially cheaper therapeutic option. One analysis, in a Canadian context and using data from the Three-D study, calculated a saving of $2451 per remission achieved with TBS versus standard rTMS [39].

It is worthy of note, however, that although the efficacy of TBS has been established through at least one substantial noninferiority study, it has not been demonstrated in any form of large multisite sham-controlled clinical trial in the same way that the effectiveness of rTMS has been confirmed.

Standard iTBS Protocol Utilized in the Three-D Study

- Left DLPFC target
- Three pulse bursts at 50 Hz
- Repeated at 5 Hz
- Trains of 2-s duration
- 8-s intertrain interval
- Total pulse number: 600

9.7 Clinical Recommendation

Notwithstanding the fact that there is somewhat less evidence supporting the use of TBS as an antidepressant treatment compared to standard forms of rTMS, it seems reasonable now to offer this as a treatment alternative for patients with major depressive disorder in clinical practice. While we await further evidence and studies exploring the possible use of accelerated forms of TBS, and a better understanding of dose in terms of the number of pulses and intensity of stimulation, adopting the approach used in the Three-D study would seem to be most clinically appropriate given that this has shown noninferiority to standard TMS in a large multisite trial (see Box).

References

1. Chung SW, Hoy KE, Fitzgerald PB (2015) Theta-burst stimulation: a new form of TMS treatment for depression? Depress Anxiety 32(3):182–192
2. Huang Y, Rothwell J (2004) The effect of short-duration bursts of high-frequency, low-intensity transcranial magnetic stimulation on the human motor cortex. Clin Neurophysiol 115:1069–1075
3. Brownjohn PW, Reynolds JN, Matheson N, Fox J, Shemmell JB (2014) The effects of individualized theta burst stimulation on the excitability of the human motor system. Brain Stimul 7(2):260–268
4. Gentner R, Wankerl K, Reinsberger C, Zeller D, Classen J (2008) Depression of human corticospinal excitability induced by magnetic theta-burst stimulation: evidence of rapid polarity-reversing metaplasticity. Cereb Cortex 18(9):2046–2053
5. Suppa A, Huang YZ, Funke K, Ridding MC, Cheeran B, Di Lazzaro V et al (2016) Ten years of theta burst stimulation in humans: established knowledge, unknowns and prospects. Brain Stimul 9(3):323–335
6. Suppa A, Ortu E, Zafar N, Deriu F, Paulus W, Berardelli A et al (2008) Theta burst stimulation induces after-effects on contralateral primary motor cortex excitability in humans. J Physiol 586(18):4489–4500
7. Paulus W (2005) Toward establishing a therapeutic window for rTMS by theta burst stimulation. Neuron 45(2):181–183
8. Gamboa OL, Antal A, Moliadze V, Paulus W (2010) Simply longer is not better: reversal of theta burst after-effect with prolonged stimulation. Exp Brain Res 204(2):181–187
9. Gamboa OLAA, Moliadze V, Paulus W (2010) Simply longer is not better: reversal of theta burst after-effect with prolonged stimulation. Exp Brain Res 204(2):181–187
10. Chung SW, Lewis BP, Rogasch NC, Saeki T, Thomson RH, Hoy KE et al (2017) Demonstration of short-term plasticity in the dorsolateral prefrontal cortex with theta burst stimulation: a TMS-EEG study. Clin Neurophysiol 128(7):1117–1126
11. Chung SW, Rogasch NC, Hoy KE, Fitzgerald PB (2018) The effect of single and repeated prefrontal intermittent theta burst stimulation on cortical reactivity and working memory. Brain Stimul 11(3):566–574
12. Chung SW, Rogasch NC, Hoy KE, Sullivan CM, Cash RFH, Fitzgerald PB (2018) Impact of different intensities of intermittent theta burst stimulation on the cortical properties during TMS-EEG and working memory performance. Hum Brain Mapp 39(2):783–802
13. Wu C-C, Tsai C-H, Lu M-K, Chen C-M, Shen W-C, Su K-P (2010) Theta-burst repetitive transcranial magnetic stimulation for treatment-resistant obsessive-compulsive disorder with concomitant depression. J Clin Psychiatry 71(4):504–506

14. Agnew ZK, Banissy M, McGettigan C, Walsh V, Scott SK (2018) Investigating the neural basis of theta burst stimulation to premotor cortex on emotional vocalization perception: a combined TMS-fMRI study. Front Hum Neurosci 12:150
15. Cardenas-Morales LGG, Kammer T (2010) Exploring the after-effects of theta burst magnetic stimulation on the human motor cortex: a functional imaging study. Hum Brain Mapp 2:1948–1960
16. Li CT, Chen MH, Juan CH, Liu RS, Lin WC, Bai YM et al (2018) Effects of prefrontal theta-burst stimulation on brain function in treatment-resistant depression: a randomized sham-controlled neuroimaging study. Brain Stimul 11(5):1054–1062
17. Mochizuki H, Furubayashi T, Hanajima R, Terao Y, Mizuno Y, Okabe S et al (2007) Hemoglobin concentration changes in the contralateral hemisphere during and after theta burst stimulation of the human sensorimotor cortices. Exp Brain Res 180(4):667–675
18. Tupak SV, Dresler T, Badewien M, Hahn T, Ernst LH, Herrmann MJ et al (2013) Inhibitory transcranial magnetic theta burst stimulation attenuates prefrontal cortex oxygenation. Hum Brain Mapp 34(1):150–157
19. Holzer M, Padberg F (2010) Intermittent theta burst stimulation (iTBS) ameliorates therapy-resistant depression: a case series. Brain Stimul 3(3):181–183
20. Chistyakov AV, Rubicsek O, Kaplan B, Zaaroor M, Klein E (2010) Safety, tolerability and preliminary evidence for antidepressant efficacy of theta-burst transcranial magnetic stimulation in patients with major depression. Int J Neuropsychopharmacol 13(3):387–393
21. Beynel L, Chauvin A, Guyader N, Harquel S, Szekely D, Bougerol T et al (2014) What saccadic eye movements tell us about TMS-induced neuromodulation of the DLPFC and mood changes: a pilot study in bipolar disorders. Front Integr Neurosci 8:65
22. Chistyakov AV, Kreinin B, Marmor S, Kaplan B, Khatib A, Darawsheh N et al (2015) Preliminary assessment of the therapeutic efficacy of continuous theta-burst magnetic stimulation (cTBS) in major depression: a double-blind sham-controlled study. J Affect Disord 170:225–229
23. Duprat R, Desmyter S, Rudi de R, van Heeringen K, Van den Abbeele D, Tandt H et al (2016) Accelerated intermittent theta burst stimulation treatment in medication-resistant major depression: a fast road to remission? J Affect Disord 200:6–14
24. Li CTCM, Juan CH, Huang HH, Chen LF, Hsieh JC, Tu PC, Bai YM, Tsai SJ, Lee YC, Su TP (2014) Efficacy of prefrontal theta-burst stimulation in refractory depression: a randomized sham controlled study. Brain 137:2088–2098
25. Plewnia C, Pasqualetti P, Grosse S, Schlipf S, Wasserka B, Zwissler B et al (2014) Treatment of major depression with bilateral theta burst stimulation: a randomized controlled pilot trial. J Affect Disord 156:219–223
26. Prasser J, Schecklmann M, Poeppl TB, Frank E, Kreuzer PM, Hajak G et al (2015) Bilateral prefrontal rTMS and theta burst TMS as an add-on treatment for depression: a randomized placebo controlled trial. World J Biol Psychiatry 16(1):57–65
27. Li CT, Cheng CM, Chen MH, Juan CH, Tu PC, Bai YM et al (2020) Antidepressant efficacy of prolonged intermittent theta burst stimulation monotherapy for recurrent depression and comparison of methods for coil positioning: a randomized, double-blind, sham-controlled study. Biol Psychiatry 87(5):443–450
28. Berlim MT, McGirr A, Rodrigues Dos Santos N, Tremblay S, Martins R (2017) Efficacy of theta burst stimulation (TBS) for major depression: an exploratory meta-analysis of randomized and sham-controlled trials. J Psychiatr Res 90:102–109
29. McGirr A, Vila-Rodriguez F, Cole J, Torres IJ, Arumugham SS, Keramatian K et al (2021) Efficacy of active vs sham intermittent theta burst transcranial magnetic stimulation for patients with bipolar depression: a randomized clinical trial. JAMA Netw Open 4(3):e210963
30. Blumberger DM, Vila-Rodriguez F, Thorpe KE, Feffer K, Noda Y, Giacobbe P et al (2018) Effectiveness of theta burst versus high-frequency repetitive transcranial magnetic stimulation in patients with depression (THREE-D): a randomised non-inferiority trial. Lancet 391(10131):1683–1692

31. Bakker N, Shahab S, Giacobbe P, Blumberger DM, Daskalakis ZJ, Kennedy SH et al (2015) rTMS of the dorsomedial prefrontal cortex for major depression: safety, tolerability, effectiveness, and outcome predictors for 10 Hz versus intermittent theta-burst stimulation. Brain Stimul 8(2):208–215
32. Tendler A, Sisko E, DeLuca M, Corbett-Methot S, Sutton-DeBord J, Brown J et al (2017) H1-coil intermittent theta burst stimulation for a patient with a high motor threshold: case report. Brain Stimul 10(4):e36–e37
33. Fitzgerald PB, Chen L, Richardson K, Daskalakis ZJ, Hoy KE (2020) A pilot investigation of an intensive theta burst stimulation protocol for patients with treatment resistant depression. Brain Stimul 13(1):137–144
34. Cole EJ, Stimpson KH, Bentzley BS, Gulser M, Cherian K, Tischler C et al (2020) Stanford accelerated intelligent neuromodulation therapy for treatment-resistant depression. Am J Psychiatry 177(8):716–726
35. Rachid F (2017) Safety and efficacy of theta-burst stimulation in the treatment of psychiatric disorders: a review of the literature. J Nerv Ment Dis 205(11):823–839
36. Lenoir C, Algoet M, Vanderclausen C, Peeters A, Santos SF, Mouraux A (2018) Report of one confirmed generalized seizure and one suspected partial seizure induced by deep continuous theta burst stimulation of the right operculo-insular cortex. Brain Stimul 11(5):1187–1188
37. Oberman LM, Pascual-Leone A (2009) Report of seizure induced by continuous theta burst stimulation. Brain Stimul 2(4):246–247
38. Oberman L, Edwards D, Eldaief M, Pascual-Leone A (2011) Safety of theta burst transcranial magnetic stimulation: a systematic review of the literature. J Clin Neurophysiol 28(1):67–74
39. Mendlowitz AB, Shanbour A, Downar J, Vila-Rodriguez F, Daskalakis ZJ, Isaranuwatchai W et al (2019) Implementation of intermittent theta burst stimulation compared to conventional repetitive transcranial magnetic stimulation in patients with treatment resistant depression: a cost analysis. PLoS One 14(9):e0222546

10 Accelerated and Intensive rTMS Treatment Protocols

Abstract

Accelerated and intensive TMS protocols have been developed to try and produce faster, more efficient, or more substantial antidepressant clinical responses. To date, a series of studies have explored the use of treatment provided on a twice-daily basis or in more intensive schedules, including those where a full treatment course is condensed into a week or less. Studies conducted to date suggest that these types of protocols can have antidepressant efficacy but we lack substantial large noninferiority trials, or large sham-controlled trials, that would be required to facilitate introduction of these types of schedules into clinical practice.

10.1 Introduction

One of the clinically challenging aspects of rTMS treatment is that a typical course of therapy lasts for at least 4 weeks and typically longer. This, coupled with the need for daily treatment sessions, results in significant treatment costs, considerable inconvenience for patients, and slow accumulation of clinical benefits if treatment is successful. This makes the use of TMS in the treatment of patients who need a rapid treatment response, for example, the presence of significant suicidal ideation, quite problematic.

For these reasons, there has been considerable interest in the use of rTMS protocols to try to shorten the duration of treatment required to achieve clinical benefits. Overall, these approaches have been motivated by several interacting motivations:

1. To make clinical response to rTMS therapy more rapid.
2. To reduce the number of days on which patients have to attend to therapy to make it more efficient and less costly.

P. B. Fitzgerald, Z. J. Daskalakis, *rTMS Treatment for Depression*, https://doi.org/10.1007/978-3-030-91519-3_10

3. To enhance treatment efficacy through the provision of more intensive therapy.

A number of approaches have been undertaken in the development of these accelerated or more intensive protocols. Most broadly speaking, these approaches can be categorized into those where treatment is provided twice daily and protocols that are even more intensive than this. The use of the term accelerated rTMS is often used to describe studies in this area although it tends to conflate approaches which are designed to increase the speed of treatment response with those designed to enhance efficacy or improve efficiency. Of note, accelerated trials have been conducted using low-frequency stimulation (exclusively 1 Hz), high-frequency stimulation (both 10 and 20 Hz), and theta-burst stimulation.

10.2 Twice-Daily rTMS

rTMS has been applied in twice-daily protocols mostly using high-frequency stimulation although Tor et al. described very limited antidepressant effects of what was mostly two sessions of 1 Hz stimulation applied to the right DLPFC (900 pulses per session) with a small group of 7 patients with treatment-resistant depression [1].

The first study applying two sessions of 10 Hz stimulation found only limited antidepressant benefits using two sessions (1500 pulses per session) per day for 10 treatment days [2]. Twice-daily treatment was applied in a second study including a variety of different intensities of stimulation but individual differences between intensities of stimulation were not reported [3]. Substantial treatment effects have been seen in more recent studies. For example, greater effects and therapeutic benefits were seen with twice-daily rather than once-daily rTMS than those seen with sham stimulation [4]. However, it is not possible from the study to conclude that twice-daily treatment was more effective than once daily. The patients receiving twice-daily treatment had a total dose that was twice that received by the once-daily patients invalidating this as a direct comparison.

Two retrospective studies have compared once- to twice-daily responses and described faster but not greater therapeutic response with twice-daily treatment [5, 6]. A recent open-label analysis found greater responses to a twice-daily protocol in elderly versus younger patients without safety issues arising in the older group [7]. A second open-label analysis presented data from 27 patients treated with twice-daily therapy. Thirty-seven percent of patients remitted and 56% were classified as responders [8]. Finally, a third open-label study in 24 patients reported significant antidepressant benefits but no changes on a number of decision-making and impulse control tasks [9].

One study has described the use of twice-daily TBS treatment in a group of 12 patients with bipolar depression compared to 14 receiving sham in 30 sessions applied over 15 days [10]. Response and remission rates were numerically higher in the active compared to the sham group (72% vs. 42% for response, 42% vs. 25% for remission), but these differences did not reach significance, not surprising given the small sample size.

10.2.1 Summary and Clinical Recommendations

Although studies conducted to date suggest that there are antidepressant effects of rTMS when applied on a twice-daily basis, the evidence base does not support the routine use of this form of stimulation. We lack substantial sham-controlled data or a large noninferiority study. There is no suggestion that twice-daily treatment will produce a greater clinical response than once-daily treatment if the same number of stimulation sessions is applied.

10.3 Intensive or Accelerated rTMS

An increasing number of studies are exploring the use of more intensive protocols, with these usually labeled as "accelerated." It is worthy of note, however, that there is not a lot of evidence to date that these protocols produce substantially more rapidly effective clinical response. The first of these studies provided 15 low-dose TMS sessions across a 2-day period in a group of patients who were simultaneously admitted to an inpatient program [11]. Fourteen patients were treated showing a response rate of 43% at the end of treatment and 36% at 6-week follow-up.

This study was then followed up by two crossover studies, one using standard rTMS and one using iTBS which provided supportive evidence that accelerated treatment is feasible and safe and may provide clinical benefit [12, 13] although the crossover nature of the studies makes interpretation of the results somewhat more complicated.

Several other small studies have explored forms of accelerated treatment, predominately providing information about feasibility rather than efficacy Dardenne et al. provided 20 sessions over 4 days in a group of 10 elderly subjects using 20 Hz stimulation [14]. George et al. provided 9 treatment sessions over 3 days in 20 suicidal patients with PTSD or mild traumatic brain injury (compared to 21 receiving sham stimulation) [15]. There was no overall difference in reduction suicidal ideation in the two groups although the active group appeared to have a more rapid diminution in severity of suicidal ideation.

In a significantly larger trial, we directly compared response to an intensive TMS schedule to 4 weeks/20 treatments of standard once-daily rTMS [16]. Patients in accelerated group received three sessions per day for 3 days in week 1, three sessions per day for 2 days in week 2, and one session per day for 1 day in week 3. The overall pulse number was balanced between the two groups. One hundred and twenty-five patients were randomized in this trial. There were no significant differences in overall outcome between the accelerated and standard treatment groups. Accelerated treatment, however, was not associated with a more rapid diminution of depressive symptoms.

We structured our treatment protocol, with additional treatment days in week 2 and week 3, following the conduct of two pilot studies where treatment was provided only within 1 week. In the patients in these pilot studies we saw a significant early relapse rate, motivating us to include a slightly more extended, but less intensive, component of the treatment course. At 1-month follow-up, the patients in accelerated group in the larger trial [16] did not show any evidence of a higher early relapse rate compared to those receiving 4 weeks of daily treatment.

We have more recently followed this with a study using iTBS and a similar method although the accelerated group received one further day of treatment in week 4 [17]. In a second study, patients receiving the intensive iTBS treatment improved to the same degree as that receiving 4 weeks of standard 10 Hz stimulation, although response was also not more rapid. Of note, providing iTBS in this matter was far more efficient and anecdotally more acceptable to patients.

A small number of other studies have explored the use of intensive TBS protocols. One open-label study described the provision of 20 sessions across 8 days in 9 patients with MDD reporting 5 responders to treatment [18]. A second open-label study provided 20 iTBS sessions over 5 days and reported a very high remission rate of over 90% with all 31 patients reported as having achieved remission from suicidal ideation [19]. This followed a report of the treatment of six patients by the same group, also reporting a very good response and remission rate [20]. Of note, the overall dose provided across these treatment sessions was very high and treatment was targeted with resting state fMRI.

10.4 Summary and Clinical Recommendations

There is limited but emerging data supporting the use of accelerated forms of rTMS and TBS. However, there is a dearth of significant comparative trials other than two studies which have compared rTMS or TBS to a standard course of 4 weeks of daily rTMS treatment. Neither of these studies were sufficient to establish noninferiority and to date there are no large sham-controlled trials that could provide support for widespread clinical implementation. At this stage accelerated treatment protocols should be considered experimental and be used almost exclusively in a research context.

References

1. Tor PC, Galvez V, Goldstein J, George D, Loo CK (2016) Pilot study of accelerated low-frequency right-sided transcranial magnetic stimulation for treatment-resistant depression. J ECT 32(3):180–182
2. Loo CK, Mitchell PB, McFarquhar TF, Malhi GS, Sachdev PS (2007) A sham-controlled trial of the efficacy and safety of twice-daily rTMS in major depression. Psychol Med 37(3):341–349
3. Szuba MP, O'Reardon JP, Rai AS, Snyder-Kastenberg J, Amsterdam JD, Gettes DR et al (2001) Acute mood and thyroid stimulating hormone effects of transcranial magnetic stimulation in major depression. Biol Psychiatry 50(1):22–27
4. Theleritis C, Sakkas P, Paparrigopoulos T, Vitoratou S, Tzavara C, Bonaccorso S et al (2017) Two versus one high-frequency repetitive transcranial magnetic stimulation session per day for treatment-resistant depression: a randomized sham-controlled trial. J ECT 33(3):190–197

5. Modirrousta M, Meek BP, Wikstrom SL (2018) Efficacy of twice-daily vs once-daily sessions of repetitive transcranial magnetic stimulation in the treatment of major depressive disorder: a retrospective study. Neuropsychiatr Dis Treat 14:309–316
6. Schulze L, Feffer K, Lozano C, Giacobbe P, Daskalakis ZJ, Blumberger DM et al (2018) Number of pulses or number of sessions? An open-label study of trajectories of improvement for once-vs. twice-daily dorsomedial prefrontal rTMS in major depression. Brain Stimul 11(2):327–336
7. Desbeaumes Jodoin V, Miron JP, Lesperance P (2019) Safety and efficacy of accelerated repetitive transcranial magnetic stimulation protocol in elderly depressed unipolar and bipolar patients. Am J Geriatr Psychiatry 27(5):548–558
8. McGirr A, Van den Eynde F, Tovar-Perdomo S, Fleck MP, Berlim MT (2015) Effectiveness and acceptability of accelerated repetitive transcranial magnetic stimulation (rTMS) for treatment-resistant major depressive disorder: an open label trial. J Affect Disord 173:216–220
9. Tovar-Perdomo S, McGirr A, Van den Eynde F, Rodrigues Dos Santos N, Berlim MT (2017) High frequency repetitive transcranial magnetic stimulation treatment for major depression: dissociated effects on psychopathology and neurocognition. J Affect Disord 217:112–117
10. Bulteau S, Beynel L, Marendaz C, Dall'Igna G, Pere M, Harquel S et al (2019) Twice-daily neuronavigated intermittent theta burst stimulation for bipolar depression: a randomized sham-controlled pilot study. Neurophysiol Clin 49(5):371–375
11. Holtzheimer PE III, McDonald WM, Mufti M, Kelley ME, Quinn S, Corso G et al (2010) Accelerated repetitive transcranial magnetic stimulation for treatment-resistant depression. Depress Anxiety 27(10):960–963
12. Baeken C, Vanderhasselt MA, Remue J, Herremans S, Vanderbruggen N, Zeeuws D et al (2013) Intensive HF-rTMS treatment in refractory medication-resistant unipolar depressed patients. J Affect Disord 151(2):625–631
13. Desmyter S, Duprat R, Baeken C, Van Autreve S, Audenaert K, van Heeringen K (2016) Accelerated intermittent theta burst stimulation for suicide risk in therapy-resistant depressed patients: a randomized, sham-controlled trial. Front Hum Neurosci 10:480
14. Dardenne A, Baeken C, Crunelle CL, Bervoets C, Matthys F, Herremans SC (2018) Accelerated HF-rTMS in the elderly depressed: a feasibility study. Brain Stimul 11(1):247–248
15. George MS, Raman R, Benedek DM, Pelic CG, Grammer GG, Stokes KT et al (2014) A two-site pilot randomized 3 day trial of high dose left prefrontal repetitive transcranial magnetic stimulation (rTMS) for suicidal inpatients. Brain Stimul 7(3):421–431
16. Fitzgerald PB, Hoy KE, Elliot D, Susan McQueen RN, Wambeek LE, Daskalakis ZJ (2018) Accelerated repetitive transcranial magnetic stimulation in the treatment of depression. Neuropsychopharmacology 43(7):1565–1572
17. Fitzgerald PB, Chen L, Richardson K, Daskalakis ZJ, Hoy KE (2020) A pilot investigation of an intensive theta burst stimulation protocol for patients with treatment resistant depression. Brain Stimul 13(1):137–144
18. Brocker E, van den Heuvel L, Seedat S (2019) Accelerated theta-burst repetitive transcranial magnetic stimulation for depression in South Africa. S Afr J Psychiatry 25:1346
19. Cole E, Stimpson K, Bentzley B, Gulser M, Cherian K, Tischler C et al (2019) Stanford accelerated intelligent neuromodulation therapy for treatment-resistant depression (SAINT-TRD). Brain Stimul 12(2):402
20. Williams N, Sudheimer K, Bentzley B, Pannu J, Stimpson K, Duvio D et al (2018) High-dose spaced theta-burst TMS as a rapid-acting antidepressant in highly refractory depression. Brain 141(3):e18

Localization and Targeting of rTMS Treatment of Depression

11

Abstract

rTMS therapy of depression typically involves stimulation of the dorsolateral prefrontal cortex (DLPFC), most commonly on the left. There are, however, a variety of methods that have been developed over time for localization of the DLPFC and the actual target within it. It is important to consider the actual target that is the focus for treatment, the method that is used to ensure accurate stimulation of the target, as well as the processes to ensure that the TMS coil remains in place, providing accurate stimulation, throughout treatment. The Beam F3 and modified 5–6 cm rule are the most common methods used in clinical practice for coil localization, but there is increasing interest in the use of neuronavigational tools based upon brain structure as well as resting state functional magnetic resonance imaging.

11.1 Introduction

The vast majority of clinical trials conducted with rTMS have utilized a relatively simplistic method for localizing the dorsolateral prefrontal cortex (DLPFC). This method involves localizing the motor cortical site for hand muscles and then measuring 5 cm anterior in a parasagittal line over the scalp surface (5 cm method) (see Chap. 12) [1]. However, research has demonstrated that this is likely to be inaccurate in a significant percentage of patients [2]: in fact, a majority of patients may not receive stimulation in true DLPFC using this approach.

Several other localization alternatives are possible, most using various forms of neuronavigation. Neuronavigational techniques most typically require the co-registration of the location of an individual's head to some form of digitized brain scan. Several hardware approaches to this form of co-registration are available which track the location of the head in three-dimensional space using either

P. B. Fitzgerald, Z. J. Daskalakis, *rTMS Treatment for Depression*, https://doi.org/10.1007/978-3-030-91519-3_11

magnetic fields, infrared, or other forms of optical localization. The procedure is undertaken whereby an individual's head in three-dimensional space is co-registered to a previously obtained brain scan, usually an MRI. The hardware is then used to localize a site on the scalp surface that corresponds to the location on the MRI scan that the operator wishes to target for rTMS treatment.

Although research is clearly indicated that the 5 cm method is suboptimal for the targeting of rTMS stimulation to the DLPFC, few studies have directly investigated the value of alternative approaches. One factor that restricts this capacity is knowing exactly where in the DLPFC one should actually target stimulation (Box 11.1). In fact, there are several quite distinct considerations in developing a targeting strategy:

1. What is the optimal target for treatment?
2. How do we ensure that the coil is accurately placed in this target?
3. How do we ensure that the coil remains consistently targeting this site during sessions and across multiple sessions?

Box 11.1 rTMS Treatment Targets in DLPFC

- Generic DLPFC
- Anatomical localization
  - Coordinate based
  - Junction of BA9 and BA 46
  - Middle third of middle frontal gyrus
  - Boundary between middle and anterior third of middle frontal gyrus
- Functional localization
  - Location of abnormal metabolism or blood flow on PET or SPECT imaging
  - Connectivity-based targeting—site of strongest anti-correlation with subgenual anterior cingulate cortex on resting state fMRI scanning
  - Targeting of functional circuitry: for example, frontal part of executive/cortical control network

11.2 Selection of a Stimulation Target

The original TMS stimulation target for studies in depression first developed in the mid-1990s was the left prefrontal cortex. It was proposed that the 5 cm method would result primarily in stimulation of the DLPFC typically considered to be represented by Brodmann areas (BA) 46 and 9 [3, 4]. This region of the brain was suggested through neuroimaging studies using techniques such as single-photon emission computed tomography (SPECT) and positron emission tomography (PET) studies [5, 6] which demonstrated abnormalities in perfusion or metabolism that appeared in depression regardless of the underlying cause and that resolved or reduced with successful therapy. There also appeared to be an association between the severity of frontal hypometabolism and depression symptom severity [6].

In reality, however, PET and SPECT studies have limited anatomical resolution and did not really provide a specific treatment target, certainly not at the level of defining a subregion of the DLPFC itself which is actually anatomically quite large.

In regard to structural neuroanatomy, the boundaries of the DLPFC were originally described by Brodmann during the dissection of a single brain in the 1900s (areas 9 and 46). These regions are relatively expansive across the superior, middle, and inferior frontal gyri. A more recent redefinition of areas 9 and 46 based on the dissection of multiple brains produced a more narrowly defined area [7]. In this redefinition, area 9 is predominately contained within the superior frontal gyrus across an expanse of approximately 2.5 cm. Area 46 is localized over the middle portion of the middle frontal gyrus with an anterior-posterior extension of approximately 2 cm. However, the total volume of the DLPFC based on this more restricted definition still exceeds the area that is likely to be stimulated by standard figure-of-eight TMS coils.

11.2.1 Anatomical Localization

The approach that has been most considered from a purely anatomical perspective has been to try to target something approximating the junction of BA 9 and 46 based upon this more restricted definition which should produce stimulation of a significant proportion of the DLPFC as defined in this way. As such, one would use a structural MRI scan and a specific coordinate system or anatomical landmarks. The latter approach would place the stimulation coil such that it would ensure some degree of meaningful stimulation of both of these regions.

One previous study has specifically used this approach to target a coordinate-based localization (Talairach coordinates −45, 45, 35) and demonstrated that stimulation of this site appeared to produce greater antidepressant effects than those produced with stimulation using the 5 cm method [8].

An approach using anatomical landmarks to locate the approximate junction of BA9 and BA46 on MRI images has also been developed and adopted in one commercially available neuronavigation-based TMS system [9]. An approach like this was tested in a recent trial which compared treatment targeted to the junction between the middle and anterior third of the middle frontal gyrus to treatment targeted to the F3 EEG location [10]. This trial did not demonstrate significant differences between targeted and nontargeted treatments although there are a number of factors that this could be attributed to. First, treatment was provided on an inpatient basis when there was likely to be strong nonspecific effects across the groups. Perhaps more importantly, using the F3 EEG localization method is the control condition likely to have meant that there would be little variation between the treatment sites targeted in the two groups. This notion is supported by the subanalyses reported that was no difference in the assessed e-field at the neuronavigational target region between the two groups, resulting in considerable overlap in the effects of stimulation at the two treatment sites.

11.2.2 Functional Localization

In addition to this approach of targeting the junction between BA9 and BA 46, a number of lines of research have attempted to explore whether a specific target may be identified within the DLPFC that may prove to be a better alternative. Given that the DLPFC is a relatively extensive area, a second neuronavigational approach would be to target stimulation based on knowledge from functional imaging of the regions within the DLPFC that are known to be abnormally active in depressive states. A considerable range of functional neuroimaging studies using positron emission tomography (PET) and functional magnetic resonance imaging (fMRI) have explored brain regions involved in depression: regions that change with successful medication treatment and regions activated by various emotional and cognitive tasks. Unfortunately, these studies have produced a relatively diverse range of results that are somewhat hard to integrate.

In an attempt to synthesize some of these results in a way that would be useful for considering a treatment target, we conducted several meta-analytic studies grouping the results of studies conducted with diverse methodologies (including resting studies, studies of the effect of antidepressant treatment and of emotional or cognitive task induction) to try and establish a consistent or common stimulation target [11, 12]. We found a number of clusters in the DLPFC of both the left and right hemispheres. The largest cluster identified—actually an increase in activity with successful antidepressant medication treatment—was located relatively posterior in the left DLPFC (centered at Talairach coordinates −36, 18, 32). This is reasonably consistent with the area of the DLPFC which would traditionally be targeted using the 5 cm method. One study localizing this 5 cm site identified the equivalent coordinates as −40, 18, and 49 (converted from MNI coordinates in [13]).

Several studies have attempted to target treatment based upon areas of hypometabolism on PET scanning [14, 15]. These studies have generally not found an improved treatment response based on PET metabolism data although [15] did support the notion of targeting the DLPFC based on structural neuroimaging.

An alternative approach using neuroimaging involves the analysis of functional imaging data, this time using connectivity analysis of resting state functional MRI data. This approach, developed by Fox and colleagues, is based on the use of connectivity analysis to identify the region in the DLPFC that is most strongly anti-correlated with activity in the subgenual anterior cingulate cortex (SGACC) [13]. This line of research began by identifying the location of strongest anti-correlation found in a group of subjects and then exploring how this location related to the site is utilized in a variety of rTMS depression studies [13, 16]. This analysis found a positive relationship between how close the site of stimulation was to the proposed "optimal" anti-correlated stimulation location and clinical outcomes with rTMS treatment. Subsequently, this relationship has been replicated in an independent cohort [17]. Specifically, antidepressant efficacy of rTMS treatment was significantly related to DLPFC-SGACC connectivity when using functional connectivity maps from a group of depressed patients or a large group of healthy individuals. In addition, in this study, there was a stronger relationship between treatment response and connectivity when the latter was calculated through the analysis of each patient's individual connectivity-related stimulation site than when a group average stimulation site was used. An individualized approach using these methods was adopted in a recent trial of accelerated theta-burst stimulation which reported very high clinical response rates, but given that there were multiple novel features in this protocol, it is challenging to know if the targeting method contributed to the excellent outcomes seen [18].

It is of significance to note that the stimulation site identified in these connectivity-based studies tends to be significantly more anterior and more lateral than the stimulation site identified with the 5 cm method or other targeting approaches. This finding is consistent with one previous study, investigating the relationship between clinical response and coil location, which had suggested that a more anterior and lateral location was associated with a greater degree of clinical response [19] and a second study which reported poor outcomes with the most posterior coil locations in a large randomized trial [20].

11.3 Is There Just One Optimal Target?

Although much of this research is predicated on the idea that there is an optimal treatment target, either at a group or an individual patient level, it may well be the case that there is more than one potential optimal site. One recent study which analyzed several MRI and clinical datasets to explore the relationship between the changes induced with rTMS and specific symptoms of depression and the patterns of functional imaging changes seen with connectivity analysis [21] found two discrete clusters of depressive symptoms where improvement in these symptom groups was related to stimulation at two quite separate stimulation targets.

In regard to these two clusters, one cluster of symptoms was labeled "dysphoric," and this group of symptoms responded best when TMS stimulation was applied at a quite anterior-lateral target close to that seen in the previously discussed DLPFC-SGACC connectivity studies. The second group of symptoms, labeled as "anxiosomatic"—consisting predominantly of anxiety and somatic symptoms—improved with stimulation at a much more posterior and somewhat more medial site, much closer to where one would expect to be stimulating with treatment localized using the 5 cm method.

It is possible, based upon this analysis, that response rates in different clinical trials using different targets have been driven by targeting at these two sites. Specifically, early trials targeting the 5 cm method would have resulted in significant improvement in the so-called anxiosomatic symptoms, whereas more recent trials targeting the anterior localized sites may be improving more of the dysphoric symptom clusters.

As such, each targeting approach may be just producing optimal stimulation in a subgroup of patients. Some support from this notion comes from studies which have looked at the variability in the optimal site of DLPFC-SGACC connectivity seen between individuals [22]. A recent analysis found that the optimal DLPFC-SGACC connectivity-based stimulation target for individual subjects was considerably variable across the DLPFC with subjects having optimal locations across both the more posterior and anterior regions identified by Siddiqi et al. [21]. It may well be that treatment responses have remained modest, regardless of treatment target, because with any one non-personalized target, be it more posterior or anterior, only a subgroup of patients is receiving optimal stimulation.

11.4 How Do We Localize Treatment to the DLPFC?

As summarized in Table 11.1, there are now a variety of means of localization of the TMS coil to whatever target is chosen for treatment. The first approach to stimulation localization was the so-called 5 cm method, which was used in the initial rTMS depression studies and most studies through until the late 2000s, including the pivotal Neuronetics study leading to device approval in the USA and eventually in many other countries (Box 11.2). However, it was recognized fairly early on in the development of rTMS methods that this approach would result in localization to a quite posterior location relative to the DLPFC and, in many patient treatments, to the premotor, rather than dorsolateral prefrontal, cortex. As

Table 11.1 Pros and cons of various methods for coil localization

Method	Pros	Cons
5 cm method	Used in many studies including Neuronetics pivotal trial Simple and inexpensive	Fails to localize to true DLPFC in many subjects
6 or 7 cm method	Used in multisite and smaller trials Simple, cheap	Lack of clear standardization if varied from patient to patient
EEG-based F3 location (cap or measured)	Inexpensive	Lack of clarity in what F3 targets and potentially inconsistent
Beam F3	Inexpensive Anterior target close to optimal site for DLPFC-SGACC connectivity	Not used in most efficacy trials
Neuronavigation based	Most accurate method	Lack of clarity on best target Costly and more complex

noted above, several studies have subsequently suggested that a more anterior stimulation target (and perhaps more lateral) would be more likely to produce effective response [19, 20].

Box 11.2 Six Centimeter Method for Location of rTMS Treatment Site

1. Locate the cortical site for optimal stimulation of hand muscles in the contralateral side.
2. Mark this site on the scalp.
3. Using a flexible measuring tape, measure 6 cm forward (or more as defined by protocol) from the motor site in a sagittal plane (see Fig. 11.1).
4. Mark the subsequent site.

Measuring the distance between this site and several anatomical landmarks (e.g., the preauricular and nasion points) will allow the re-measurement of this site without the localization of the RMT on subsequent days (Fig. 11.2).

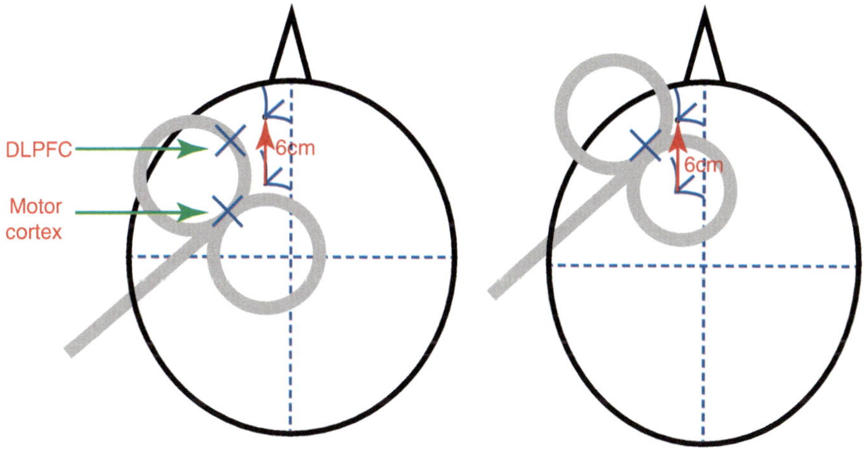

Fig. 11.1 Moving the coil forward 6 cm from the motor cortex to the DLPFC

As such, from the late 2000s attempts began to modify the 5 cm method to produce more consistent DLPFC localization. The simplest version of this was to move the coil a little bit further forward: perhaps 5 1/2, 6, or even 7 cm. However, all variations of this approach fail to take differences in head size into account resulting in what is likely to be some degree of systematic inconsistency in targeting between individuals.

Therefore, approaches were developed which would take variations in head size into account, typically based upon EEG electrode measurements. Specifically, localizing treatment to the site of the F3 EEG electrode was thought likely to result

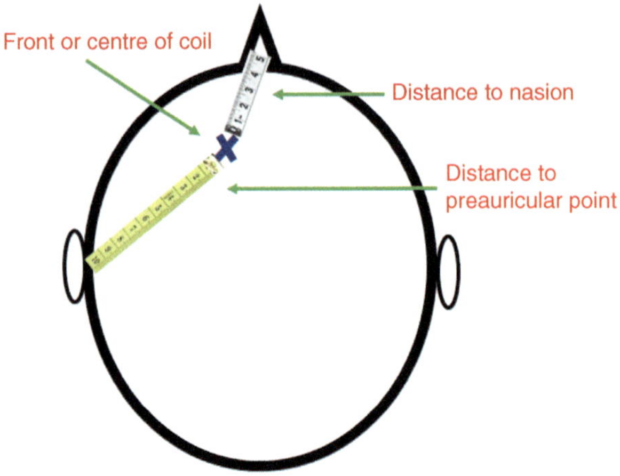

Fig. 11.2 Using measurements to the nasion and preauricular point to localize the front or center of the TMS coil

in relatively accurate stimulation of the DLPFC. This can be done by placing an EEG cap on the head to find the location of the F3 electrode side, or by following a standard set of measurements which are typically used to localize EEG electrode when they are attached to the scalp without a cap.

Several studies have explored the location of cortical stimulation that results from this type of approach. As we have recently demonstrated, these have actually found a fairly variable set of scalp or cortical coordinates between studies. It is reasonable to assume that relatively small differences in EEG localization techniques (and perhaps in the methods used to map cortical locations) have resulted in significant differences in cortical localization. These studies have reported cortical stimulation locations that spread several centimeters across the DLPFC.

An alternative and more efficient approach is the so-called Beam F3 method. The Beam F3 approach uses a simpler set of measurements of head size (tragus to tragus, nasion to inion and head circumference) entered into an algorithm that is available on the Internet, to generate two numbers used to localize the treatment site. These are a specific distance along the front of the head, to the left, in the circumference from the midline directly above the nasion (point X), and the distance from vertex toward point X (see Fig. 11.3).

Studies investigating the cortical location localized using the Beam F3 approach tend to suggest that it results in treatment at a fairly anterior site, close to that identified with the resting state fMRI connectivity approach and with the Talairach coordinates −45, 45, and 35 (ref). In fact, the Beam F3 site is much more anterior than that localized via the 5 cm method (or limited variations). Trapp et al. found a mean 2.6 ± 1.0 cm anterolateral distance between Beam F3 and 5.5 cm identified sites [23]. Of perhaps equal significance, there was less variability in the application of the site identified with the Beam F3 approach and less inter-operator variability in the resultant site localization.

The most superficially appealing approaches are those using neuronavigational techniques with either structural or functional MRI data, to establish the treatment target, as they allow for certainty about the actual targeted site, rather than having this be inferred from other research (Box 11.3). Studies have shown that they do produce greater consistency of location to a stimulation site [24]. They, however, are more time consuming, require patients to typically undergo an expensive MRI scan, and involve the application of equipment that can be expensive and complicated to operate.

Box 11.3 Neuronavigational Coil Localization

A number of systems are commercially available for the neuronavigational localization of TMS stimulation, although some of these have been predominately developed for research applications and are not necessarily set up for easy translational use in clinical practice. All of these systems typically map the position of the head (and hence the brain) to a reference MRI image. Once this mapping has occurred, the software will represent the relationship of a sensor, or TMS equipment that the sensor is attached to, to the MRI image of the brain. This allows the user to identify accurately where the TMS coil is to be placed in reference to the brain scan rather than just the scalp surface. Some systems will then allow for the position of the coil and its orientation to be tracked during stimulation (see Fig. 11.3).

One final approach that has been proposed recently for establishing the optimal target site on an individual subject level is called neuro-cardiac-guided TMS (NCG-TMS). It is based on a hypothesis that the optimal site of stimulation in the DLPFC will produce changes in parasympathetic nervous system activity resulting in changes in heart rate [25]. The first study to investigate this hypothesis provided trains of 10 Hz stimulation across seven regions in the DLPFC and studied the relationship between stimulation at these sites and changes in heart rate [26]. The two interesting findings from this study were that (1) the most common effects were seen at F3/F4 for EEG sites and (2) there was significant variation between subjects in their optimal stimulation location. There has been partial replication of these

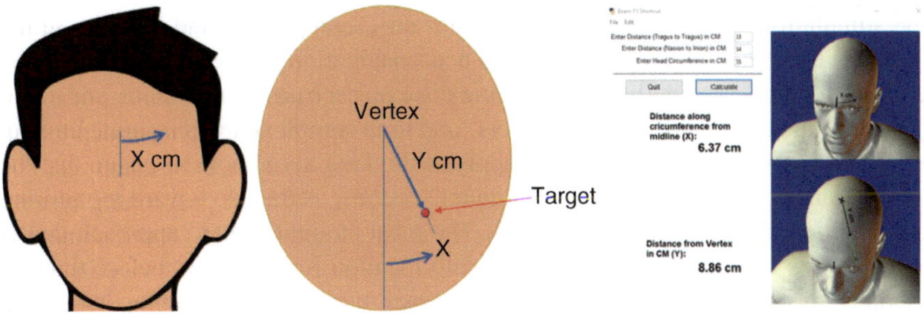

Fig. 11.3 The coordinates/numbers generated from the Beam F3 approach

results [27], but the approach needs to be more substantially and prospectively evaluated before it gets adopted into clinical practice.

11.5 How Do We Keep the Coil at the Target?

Alongside the questions of where we should target and how do we ensure the coil-induced field stimulates the target, it is worth asking the question of how do we ensure that there is consistency of stimulation of the target during an individual treatment session and across the course of multiple treatment sessions. The most simplistic way that is used to monitor the position of a stimulation coil within treatment session is to mark the front of the stimulation coil and to visibly check that the coil remains in the right place throughout the treatment. This will, however, involve the treater repeatedly approaching the patient to visibly do this, and/or engaging the patient in reporting whether they feel there has been any movement of the head relative to the stimulation coil. This might be easier to do if the position is marked on some form so that the actual mark is more readily visible than it might be through hair. The head is also a lot less likely to move, relative to the stimulation coil, if it is fully supported such that the head is unlikely to move side to side, by an appropriate series of pillows or cushions. Some TMS coil systems come with a counter pad to support the head on the opposite side from the coil such that any pressure from the coil is countered, preventing the head from moving away from the coil itself.

Several alternative approaches have been developed, predominately by equipment manufacturers. For example, the system that is embedded with the Neuronetics TMS device involves the use of a paper tape that is attached to the forehead and to the stimulation coil to ensure that there is minimal movement during stimulation but that the patient could forcibly move the head away from the coil for some reason that was necessary.

The most sophisticated mechanism to monitor coil position is the use of neuronavigation throughout the treatment session. In this way, the position of the coil, or the induced electrical field, is constantly monitored relative to the proposed stimulation target. Some neuronavigation systems come with the capacity to switch off if the stimulation field moves away from the treatment target by a predetermined distance. Clearly this sort of approach is likely to produce a very consistent location of the stimulation site but will come at greater cost, complexity, and time for setup. These will be mitigated considerably if neuronavigation is already being used for coil localization, especially if this is being done on each day of treatment, and under those circumstances, the additional "cost" and time complexity will be quite limited.

Some of the same considerations apply to thinking about how to ensure that the appropriate site is targeted across treatment sessions, as they do toward monitoring coil position within treatment sessions. The most straightforward approach that is taken in this regard is to establish the scalp location for treatment before the first therapeutic session and establish some measures, typically very simple, that can be used to ensure that the coil can be placed back at the same site each day. For example, measurements can be taken from the front of the coil to the nasion and the

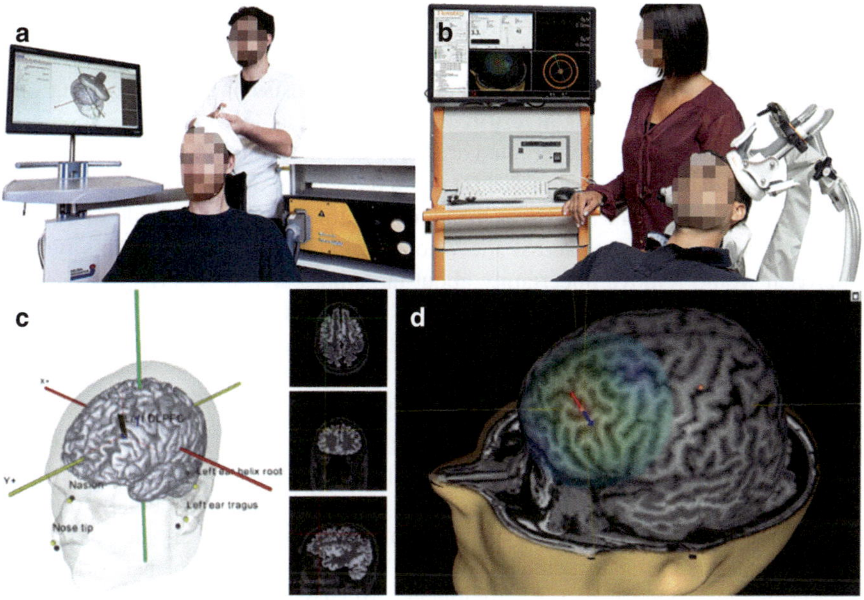

Fig. 11.4 Illustration of the equipment and interface for two neuronavigation systems, the Brain Science Tools Neuronavigator (panels **a** and **c**) and the Nexstim NBT® Navigated Brain Therapy System (panels **b** and **d**)

preauricular point. Then, when a patient returns for treatment, these two distances are remeasured to localize the front of the coil (Fig. 11.4). The same approach can be used to localize and mark the center of the stimulation coil, and there are probably advantages to measuring and marking both sites to ensure that there is some consistency in the orientation of the coil relative to the midline as well as the actual location itself.

The other systems described above can also be used to reposition the coil day by day. The Neuronetics system is set up such that the operator records several numbers when the coil is first located to the DLPFC. A fairly elaborate process is followed to realign the coil and using these numbers ensures repositioning of the coil to the same stimulation site. Neuronavigation clearly can be used for the same purpose.

Despite the lengths that we can go to ensure this consistency of stimulation, no research has really established that it is likely to produce optimal outcomes. Given the lack of certainty around understanding the optimal treatment target for rTMS in depression, one could make an argument that some variability in stimulation location around the DLPFC could actually produce better clinical better effects than treatment always being provided to exactly the same site. In the absence of meaningful research, this remains an empirical question. It is probably reasonable to reassure patients that if their experience of rTMS feels slightly different day by day, this may be of limited importance. They should certainly report to the operator if there is a significant difference in what their stimulation feels like; the methods described may be vulnerable to operator error resulting in incorrect localization.

11.6 Is Being Highly Targeted Optimal?

Related to the question of whether we should be consistent in our targeting of a particular stimulation site is a very relevant question as to whether we should be concerned with being highly targeted at all. An alternative to the search for increasingly sophisticated and fine-grained treatment targets, or more personalized targets which vary from patient to patient, is the notion that we could provide more non-focal stimulation, perhaps across the whole DLPFC, to all patients. This type of approach would remove uncertainty about targeting but would perhaps come at a cost of the stimulation of areas of the brain that are directly involved in depression itself. We then need to ask whether this collateral stimulation could result in any significant adverse consequences.

rTMS methods appear to be extraordinarily safe across their application to many areas of the brain in patient populations and in the vast number of studies that have been conducted in healthy individuals. It is possible, however, that stimulation of surrounding areas of the brain could produce side effects or could actually mitigate the therapeutic benefits to be achieved by stimulation of the primary site. For example, if we were trying to activate areas of the cognitive control network in the DLPFC but also at the same time stimulated cortical projections of the default mode network, the latter might mitigate the therapeutic effects of the former.

These questions have not really been addressed by systematic research but we can make some inferences as to the risks and benefit that would arise from a less focal approach from the research that has been conducted evaluating the efficacy of the Brainsway deep TMS system for the treatment of depression. The Brainsway H1 coil does produce somewhat deeper stimulation of the brain but at the same time significantly broader stimulation of more superficial layers of the cortex [28, 29]. Use of this coil is likely to produce stimulation of most, if not all, of the DLPFC, providing a useful test for the hypothesis that nontargeted stimulation may be helpful and not harmful. The results of studies exploring the use of the Brainsway system in depression, relative to standard forms of rTMS administered through a figure-of-eight coil, are somewhat promising in this regard although by no means definitive.

First, the results of the pivotal deep TMS trial do not provide evidence of greater efficacy compared to the results of trials evaluating standard forms of rTMS (see discussion in [30]). However, there is some interesting information in the only substantive comparative study published to date by Filipcic et al. [31]. This study, published independently of a device manufacturer, did not find superiority of deep TMS over standard rTMS on the primary outcome (remission rates), but some benefits on mean reduction in depressive symptoms and response rates were seen.

It seems reasonable to conclude that the broader stimulation achieved with a deep TMS coil does not mitigate the antidepressant effects achieved with non-focal stimulation. However, at this stage it also doesn't necessarily resolve the theoretical debate on whether broader stimulation is better than more focused because even if deep TMS proves to be a more effective approach, it would remain unclear whether this would be secondary to the "deep" component of the stimulation or the "broader"/ less focused aspect. There are also other differences between the application of deep TMS and standard rTMS (e.g., the use of 10 Hz for rTMS and 18 Hz for deep TMS) that could contribute to differences in the study conducted by Filipcic et al. [31].

11.7 Don't Forget About Coil Orientation

Although considerable attention has been placed on methods to ensure optimal coil localization, far less has been given to the orientation of the TMS coil when it is placed over the DLPFC and how this may be optimized to ensure the best clinical outcomes. In almost all circumstances, it is recommended that the TMS coil is oriented at 45° to the sagittal plane, with the handle pointing backward and away from the midline. Why do we use this approach? This is relatively straightforward. When TMS methods were being developed in the 1980s and early 1990s, it was established that this coil angle was optimal for stimulation of the hand area of the motor cortex in most individuals. This was of interest as the primary application of TMS at this time was in studying motor cortical physiology. The 45° angle was adopted as a standard that is applied to hundreds of physiological studies of the motor system over the following decades.

When TMS methods were developed for the treatment of depression, the motor cortex was also being stimulated to establish the RMT, and the coil was being moved forward to the DLPFC. The initial TMS operators just kept the coil at the same 45° angle when it was moved forward for depression treatment, and this approach, using the 45° angle, has remained what we do ever since (Fig. 11.1).

Does this make sense? It makes sense in part that the 45° angle is optimal in stimulation of the motor cortex and that this applies to most brains, because the neurons in this area of the cortex line up in specific directions quite reliably between individuals. Therefore, placing the coil at 45° to the midline is likely to be optimal for motor cortex stimulation in most people. However, this is unlikely to be the case in the DLPFC. There is no evidence that cortical neurons line up in the same directions in the DLPFC as they do in the motor cortex, and there is a lot less consistency in the orientation and structure of the prefrontal gyri (Fig. 11.5). Therefore, one can hypothesize that it is unlikely that a 45° angle will be optimal for stimulating the DLPFC in most patients.

In fact, the empirical research that we have certainly suggests that this hypothesis is true. Studies using e-field modeling [32, 33], as well those measuring vascular responses to TMS pulses with near-infrared spectroscopy [34], have shown that the optimal orientation of the TMS coil for stimulating the DLPFC is not 45° and most importantly is likely to vary between individual subjects. However, these methods for establishing optimal coil orientation in the DLPFC are relatively complex and have not yet been developed in a manner that allows them to be integrated smoothly into clinical practice. Therefore, we continue to utilize the 45° angle and will do so until we have a better way for determining this element of TMS practice in individual patients prior to treatment commencement.

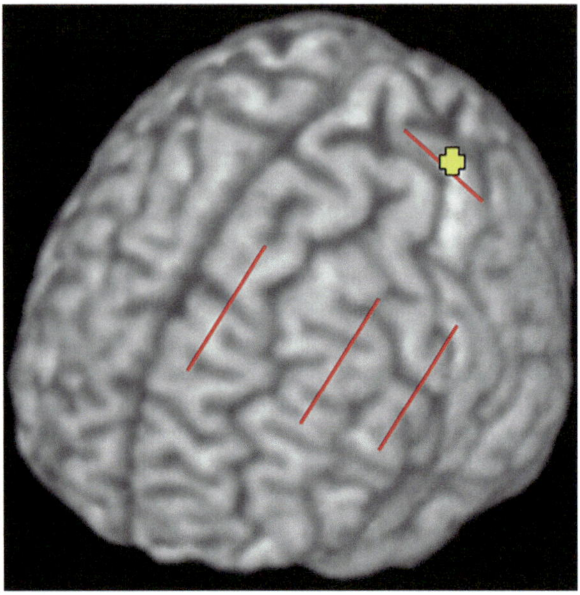

Fig. 11.5 Arrangement of gyrification. Red lines denote broad direction of gyrification. Yellow cross denotes approximate area for right thumb muscle

11.8 Clinical Application and Recommendations

As should be evident from the discussion above, there are a number of options that make sense for use in clinical practice and, at this stage, relatively sparse evidence suggesting how we should choose between these. However, this is a rapidly evolving area of TMS practice and one where the gold standard is likely to continue to evolve over the coming years. What we understand at this stage can be summarized as follows:

1. The vast majority of clinical trials demonstrating the efficacy of rTMS in depression have utilized the 5 cm method or some variation of this. However, there is relatively consistent evidence that a more anterior and somewhat more lateral treatment localization site seems to be associated with better clinical outcomes. Therefore, if using this type of method, one should at least move the coil 6 or more centimeters forward: there is reasonable evidence that 5 cm is insufficient for optimal outcomes.
2. The Beam F3 appears to be a good reliable approach to ensure consistent localization to a fairly anterior stimulation site close to what would be considered the center of the DLPFC.
3. If using a neuronavigational system and structural MRI images, the literature would support utilizing a method that localizes treatment in the region of the boundary between BA 46 and 9 as this seems to correspond reasonably well with the emerging anterior site identified through the anti-correlation studies [9].

4. The treatment coil should be oriented at 45° to the sagittal plane with the coil handle angled away from the midline although personalized methods for determining optimal coil orientation are under development.
5. In patients who are failing to respond to a particular rTMS approach, movement of the coil to an alternative location could be considered along with other forms of modification of treatment such as a switch to low-frequency right-sided rTMS or sequential bilateral rTMS (see discussion of switching options in [35] and Chap. 7).
6. Deep TMS is likely to ensure broad stimulation of the DLPFC covering multiple potential stimulation sites.

References

1. Schonfeldt-Lecuona C, Lefaucheur JP, Cardenas-Morales L, Wolf RC, Kammer T, Herwig U (2010) The value of neuronavigated rTMS for the treatment of depression. Neurophysiol Clin 40(1):37–43
2. Herwig U, Padberg F, Unger J, Spitzer M, Schonfeldt-Lecuona C (2001) Transcranial magnetic stimulation in therapy studies: examination of the reliability of "standard" coil positioning by neuronavigation. Biol Psychiatry 50(1):58–61
3. Pascual-Leone A, Rubio B, Pallardo F, Catala MD (1996) Rapid-rate transcranial magnetic stimulation of left dorsolateral prefrontal cortex in drug-resistant depression. Lancet 348(9022):233–237
4. George MS, Wasserman EM, Kimbrell TA et al (1997) Mood improvement following daily left prefrontal repetitive transcranial magnetic stimulation in patients with depression: a placebo-controlled crossover trial. Am J Psychiatry 154:1752–1756
5. George MS, Ketter TA, Post RM (1994) Prefrontal cortex dysfunction in clinical depression. Depression 2:59–72
6. George MS, Ketter TA, Post RM (1993) SPECT and PET imaging in mood disorders. J Clin Psychiatry 54(Suppl):6–13
7. Rajkowska G, Goldman-Rakic PS (1995) Cytoarchitectonic definition of prefrontal areas in the normal human cortex: II. Variability in locations of areas 9 and 46 and relationship to the Talairach Coordinate System. Cereb Cortex 5(4):323–337
8. Fitzgerald PB, Hoy K, McQueen S, Maller JJ, Herring S, Segrave R et al (2009) A randomized trial of rTMS targeted with MRI based neuro-navigation in treatment-resistant depression. Neuropsychopharmacology 34(5):1255–1262
9. Mylius V, Ayache SS, Ahdab R, Farhat WH, Zouari HG, Belke M et al (2013) Definition of DLPFC and M1 according to anatomical landmarks for navigated brain stimulation: inter-rater reliability, accuracy, and influence of gender and age. NeuroImage 78:224–232
10. Hebel T, Gollnitz A, Schoisswohl S, Weber FC, Abdelnaim M, Wetter TC et al (2021) A direct comparison of neuronavigated and non-neuronavigated intermittent theta burst stimulation in the treatment of depression. Brain Stimul 14(2):335–343
11. Fitzgerald PB, Oxley TJ, Laird AR, Kulkarni J, Egan GF, Daskalakis ZJ (2006) An analysis of functional neuroimaging studies of dorsolateral prefrontal cortical activity in depression. Psychiatry Res 148(1):33–45
12. Fitzgerald PB, Laird AR, Maller J, Daskalakis ZJ (2008) A meta-analytic study of changes in brain activation in depression. Hum Brain Mapp 29(6):683–695
13. Fox MD, Buckner RL, White MP, Greicius MD, Pascual-Leone A (2012) Efficacy of transcranial magnetic stimulation targets for depression is related to intrinsic functional connectivity with the subgenual cingulate. Biol Psychiatry 72(7):595–603

14. Herwig U, Lampe Y, Juengling FD, Wunderlich A, Walter H, Spitzer M et al (2003) Add-on rTMS for treatment of depression: a pilot study using stereotaxic coil-navigation according to PET data. J Psychiatr Res 37(4):267–275
15. Paillere Martinot ML, Galinowski A, Ringuenet D, Gallarda T, Lefaucheur JP, Bellivier F et al (2010) Influence of prefrontal target region on the efficacy of repetitive transcranial magnetic stimulation in patients with medication-resistant depression: a [(18)F]-fluorodeoxyglucose PET and MRI study. Int J Neuropsychopharmacol 13(1):45–59
16. Weigand A, Horn A, Caballero R, Cooke D, Stern AP, Taylor SF et al (2018) Prospective validation that subgenual connectivity predicts antidepressant efficacy of transcranial magnetic stimulation sites. Biol Psychiatry 84(1):28–37
17. Cash RFH, Zalesky A, Thomson RH, Tian Y, Cocchi L, Fitzgerald PB (2019) Subgenual functional connectivity predicts antidepressant treatment response to transcranial magnetic stimulation: independent validation and evaluation of personalization. Biol Psychiatry 86(2):e5–e7
18. Cole EJ, Stimpson KH, Bentzley BS, Gulser M, Cherian K, Tischler C et al (2020) Stanford accelerated intelligent neuromodulation therapy for treatment-resistant depression. Am J Psychiatry 177(8):716–726
19. Herbsman T, Avery D, Ramsey D, Holtzheimer P, Wadjik C, Hardaway F et al (2009) More lateral and anterior prefrontal coil location is associated with better repetitive transcranial magnetic stimulation antidepressant response. Biol Psychiatry 66(5):509–515
20. Johnson KA, Baig M, Ramsey D, Lisanby SH, Avery D, McDonald WM et al (2013) Prefrontal rTMS for treating depression: location and intensity results from the OPT-TMS multi-site clinical trial. Brain Stimul 6(2):108–117
21. Siddiqi SH, Taylor SF, Cooke D, Pascual-Leone A, George MS, Fox MD (2020) Distinct symptom-specific treatment targets for circuit-based neuromodulation. Am J Psychiatry 177(5):435–446
22. Cash RFH, Cocchi L, Lv J, Fitzgerald PB, Zalesky A (2020) Functional magnetic resonance imaging–guided personalization of transcranial magnetic stimulation treatment for depression. JAMA Psychiatry 78(3):337–339
23. Trapp NT, Bruss J, King Johnson M, Uitermarkt BD, Garrett L, Heinzerling A et al (2020) Reliability of targeting methods in TMS for depression: beam F3 vs. 5.5 cm. Brain Stimul 13(3):578–581
24. Ahdab R, Ayache SS, Brugieres P, Goujon C, Lefaucheur JP (2010) Comparison of "standard" and "navigated" procedures of TMS coil positioning over motor, premotor and prefrontal targets in patients with chronic pain and depression. Neurophysiol Clin 40(1):27–36
25. Iseger TA, van Bueren NER, Kenemans JL, Gevirtz R, Arns M (2020) A frontal-vagal network theory for Major Depressive Disorder: implications for optimizing neuromodulation techniques. Brain Stimul 13(1):1–9
26. Iseger TA, Padberg F, Kenemans JL, Gevirtz R, Arns M (2017) Neuro-Cardiac-Guided TMS (NCG-TMS): probing DLPFC-sgACC-vagus nerve connectivity using heart rate - first results. Brain Stimul 10(5):1006–1008
27. Kaur M, Michael JA, Hoy KE, Fitzgibbon BM, Ross MS, Iseger TA et al (2020) Investigating high- and low-frequency neuro-cardiac-guided TMS for probing the frontal vagal pathway. Brain Stimul 13(3):931–938
28. Deng ZD, Lisanby SH, Peterchev AV (2013) Electric field depth-focality tradeoff in transcranial magnetic stimulation: simulation comparison of 50 coil designs. Brain Stimul 6(1):1–13
29. Guadagnin V, Parazzini M, Liorni I, Fiocchi S, Ravazzani P (2014) Modelling of deep transcranial magnetic stimulation: different coil configurations. Annu Int Conf IEEE Eng Med Biol Soc 2014:4306–4309
30. Levkovitz Y, Isserles M, Padberg F, Lisanby SH, Bystritsky A, Xia G et al (2015) Efficacy and safety of deep transcranial magnetic stimulation for major depression: a prospective multicenter randomized controlled trial. World Psychiatry 14(1):64–73
31. Filipcic I, Simunovic Filipcic I, Milovac Z, Sucic S, Gajsak T, Ivezic E et al (2019) Efficacy of repetitive transcranial magnetic stimulation using a figure-8-coil or an H1-coil in treatment of major depressive disorder; a randomized clinical trial. J Psychiatr Res 114:113–119

32. Gomez LJ, Dannhauer M, Peterchev AV (2021) Fast computational optimization of TMS coil placement for individualized electric field targeting. NeuroImage 228:117696
33. Gomez-Tames J, Hamasaka A, Laakso I, Hirata A, Ugawa Y (2018) Atlas of optimal coil orientation and position for TMS: a computational study. Brain Stimul 11(4):839–848
34. Thomson RH, Cleve TJ, Bailey NW, Rogasch NC, Maller JJ, Daskalakis ZJ et al (2013) Blood oxygenation changes modulated by coil orientation during prefrontal transcranial magnetic stimulation. Brain Stimul 6(4):576–581
35. Fitzgerald PB (2020) An update on the clinical use of repetitive transcranial magnetic stimulation in the treatment of depression. J Affect Disord 276:90–103

Treatment Intensity, the Resting Motor Threshold and rTMS Treatment Dosing

12

Abstract

The determination of stimulation intensity for the provision of rTMS treatment is almost universally done following the determination of the resting motor threshold (RMT). There are some basic techniques which are almost universally utilized in the determination of the RMT along with some significant variations in practice, especially in regard to the method for determination of the actual threshold once the hotspot for eliciting an optimal motor response from the hand has been determined. The RMT may be affected by a number of personal and clinical factors, such as prescribed medication or alcohol consumption, that must be considered in the management of a patient undergoing rTMS treatment.

12.1 Dosing and Motor Threshold

The intensity of stimulation provided during rTMS treatment is typically defined as a percentage (usually between 0 and 100%) of the total machine output provided by the rTMS device being used. The intensity for each patient is individualized; in almost all clinical settings it is typically determined relative to that individual's resting motor threshold (RMT). The RMT is an estimate of an individual's level of motor cortical excitability, established by the application of single TMS pulses to the motor cortex. The lowest stimulation intensity required to consistently induce a motor response in a peripheral muscle is determined, usually in the abductor pollicis brevis (APB) in the contralateral hand. This sets the RMT (see Box 12.2).

P. B. Fitzgerald, Z. J. Daskalakis, *rTMS Treatment for Depression*,
https://doi.org/10.1007/978-3-030-91519-3_12

12.2 Assessment of the Resting Motor Threshold (RMT)

Typically, the RMT is defined as the minimum machine stimulator intensity required to produce a pre-specified motor response. Most commonly, this is a defined number of motor twitches observed on a certain number of occasions (e.g., on three out of five or five out of ten stimulations).

The RMT is determined by a number of factors. These include intransient factors such as the distance between the stimulation coil and the cortex, and variable factors such as medication status and sleep deprivation. Critically, the resting motor threshold is also sensitively dependent on the absence of any muscle activity. If the patient has a background level of motor activity during measurement, the RMT measured is likely to be considerably lower than the true value.

The type of motor response can be assessed in one of two ways:

1. The visual observation of a muscle twitch in the contralateral hand from the site of stimulation.
2. The measurement of a motor evoked response of a specific size in the contralateral hand. This is achieved using electromyographic equipment (EMG): a significant motor response is usually defined as an EMG deviation (motor evoked potential) of greater than 50 μV peak to peak.

Assessment of the RMT with visual observation is simple and does not require the knowledge needed to set up EMG monitoring. However, EMG monitoring does give reassurance that the patient is maintaining an adequate level of muscle relaxation. In the absence of this, considerable effort should be given to ensure the patient is as relaxed as possible throughout assessment of the RMT (Box 12.1).

Box 12.1 Future Alternatives to Assessing the RMT

Of note, although the stimulation intensity is determined relative to the RMT in almost all circumstances currently, the methodology around this may well evolve over time. The RMT is a measure of cortical excitability in the motor cortex which is clearly significantly anatomically distant from the site of depression treatment stimulation in the DLPFC. It is an assumption that motor cortical excitability is likely to be relevant to the determination of the treatment parameters required for stimulation when applied to the DLPFC itself. Attempts have been made to use TMS-EEG as a way of measuring cortical excitability directly in non-motor areas such as the prefrontal cortex and to develop these techniques as a way of determining a prefrontal motor threshold. However, using TMS-EEG is typically quite complex and there are significant barriers to clinical translation of these approaches.

A second alternative method is the use of e-field modeling to determine stimulation intensity. This approach would involve the modeling of the electrical field induced by a TMS stimulus on an individual subject's MRI scan

[1]. Intensity for treatment purposes would be determined as that which produced a sufficient electrical field in the area of the brain that was regarded as being necessary for treatment effects. This might involve a certain degree of electrical field penetration into the brain or spread over the cortical surface. This approach could be paired with the optimization of coil orientation as discussed in a previous chapter [2]. However, although promising, this approach is not currently developed sufficiently to be used in clinical practice.

In the meantime, the use of the RMT as an estimate for prefrontal treatment has support from the clinical trials of rTMS depression treatment in which few safety concerns, including only minimal incidences of seizure induction, have arisen. Treatment determined by the RMT has also clearly shown sufficient efficacy to warrant widespread clinical use.

It is likely that assessment based on EMG or visual observation methods generates a similar RMT value within individuals although studies investigating this are not completely consistent [3–5]. The EMG is capable of detecting non-visible motor twitches but will only detect activity in a single muscle. This increase in sensitivity compared to visual observation is likely balanced by the fact that when visualizing muscle activity, it can be considered in one of a number of muscles. If the RMT is measured in this way, it is likely to be of similar sensitivity to the EMG method.

The RMT can potentially be quantified in several ways. As described above, one approach is to define the RMT as a minimal intensity at which a certain number of motor evoked responses are evoked out of a predetermined number of pulses: for example, the minimal intensity at which five motor responses are seen during ten stimulation pulses. However, several software algorithms have also been developed that estimate the RMT from the size and presence of motor responses at varied stimulation intensities (e.g., as used in [6, 7]), although there remains some debate about the relative advantages and disadvantages of some of these [8]. Variation in the method for measurement of the RMT does further complicate the comparison of outcomes of various clinical trials. However, improvement in RMT estimation methods is likely to restrict the variability of measurements recorded rather than the result in a systematically higher or lower threshold used for stimulation (Box 12.2).

Box 12.2 Assessment of Resting Motor Threshold (RMT): Techniques

A number of methods have been described for the estimation of the RMT. The basic procedure is presented here for measurement of the RMT and quantification using a simple counting method.

1. Place the coil with its center approximately 2 cm lateral and 5 cm anterior in a parasagittal plane from the vertex (see Fig. 12.1). This will be approximately in line with the ears.

2. Position the coil to be on an approximately 45° angle from the midline (see Fig. 6.1).
3. Place your other hand gently yet firmly on the other side of the subject's head. Take care not to press too hard with that hand, or to press down too firmly on the coil. Make sure the subject is as relaxed as possible, especially in their arms and hands.
4. Beginning with the intensity low (30–35%), commence single pulse stimulation with pulses every 3–5 s. Slowly move the coil around the estimated location of the motor cortex, applying 1 or 2 pulses at each site. Starting at a low intensity is important to help relax the subject with stimulation unlikely to cause discomfort and familiarize them with the procedure. This process can be fast tracked for subjects who have had rTMS before.
5. If no movement/twitch is observed in the contralateral hand, then the RMT for that person is higher than the current TMS output setting. Therefore, increase the output in steps of 5%, testing the response at a number of sites/scalp locations at each step.
6. If a hand and/or wrist movement is observed, then the applied intensity is close to the RMT. Test responses at a number of areas and mark the site on the scalp which appears to produce the greatest motor response. Increase the intensity to do this a little if the observed movement is not produced on each pulse.
7. With the intensity set at a level that produces a small but regular muscle twitch, establish the scalp location that produces the optimal response. To do this, test the response to 2 or 3 pulses over an imaginary grid of points surrounding the site which you have marked (see Fig. 12.2). Mark the optimal location. This mapping process typically involves moving the coil in 0.5–1 cm increments laterally and medially of the marked point to determine the optimal site of stimulation in the lateral/medial plane. Once this is done, the coil is then moved anterior and posterior to do the same thing. If the optimal position has been moved anterior or posterior from the original plane, the process is repeated moving medially and laterally.
8. Providing stimulation with pulses of approximately 0.2 Hz at the optimal location (no more frequent than one pulse every 5 s), now establish the motor threshold by your chosen method (algorithm or counting). Note, if higher frequencies of stimulation are used, this may in itself affect cortical excitability confounding RMT assessment.
9. If using a counting method, apply pulses at a slightly suprathreshold intensity: if three muscle movements are observed during five pulses (or five out of ten), consider this level above threshold and reduce the intensity by 1%. Repeat this procedure until three (or five) responses are not seen. The RMT is 1% higher than this level. The same procedure can be undertaken with EMG where a 50 μV motor evoked potential response is considered above threshold.

10. Once the motor threshold is determined, it is a good safety check to provide stimulation at 2% or 3% below threshold in an area surrounding the previously determined optimal site. If significant motor activity is induced, it may be that the optimal site was incorrectly identified and the procedure should be repeated.

Note: You may often see a thumb movement/twitch from the very first pulse at any given intensity level but then no observed movement following further stimulation: the response is typically greater to a first rather than subsequent pulse. A failure to get consistent responses indicates that you are below the RMT.

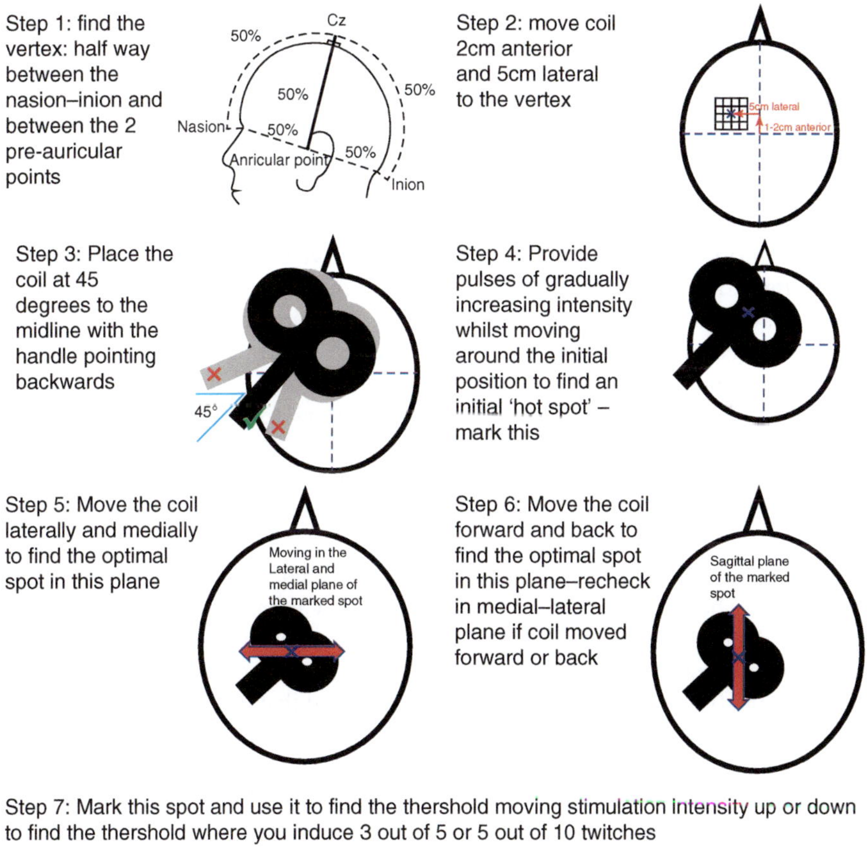

Fig. 12.1 Process of determination of the RMT. Step 1: finding the vertex. Step 2: moving the coil anterior and lateral to the vertex. Step 3: placing the coil 45° to the midline. Step 4: providing pulses of gradually increasing intensity, moving the coil around looking to evoke a motor response. Step 5: moving the coil in the medial-lateral plane. Step 6: moving the coil in the sagittal plane. Step 7: adjusting stimulation intensity to find the motor threshold

What to Do If You Are Struggling to Get an Initial Motor Response
If no response is observed when you reach between 60% and 70%, get the patient to make a tonic contraction; this slightly reduces the intensity required to produce a motor response and will help locate the spot.

For a tonic contraction, ask the participant to push their index finger against their thumb (abduction movement of the finger) and apply a small amount of tension.

If you find the hotspot to produce a motor response when making a tonic contraction, make sure to get the patient to relax to find the actual threshold.

12.3 Issues with RMT Assessment

Across time there has been considerable variation in stimulation intensity used within rTMS treatment trials for patients with depression. Initially, trials used intensities below the RMT (80–90%). However, in more recent years, trials have more typically used suprathreshold intensities of either 110% or 120%. The intensity used for stimulation has implications potentially for efficacy and definitively for safety and tolerability.

In regard to efficacy, it has been proposed that the progressive increase in stimulation intensity in treatment trials over time may have contributed to greater treatment effects in more recent studies [9]. However, a substantial number of other factors have also changed over time, including the duration of treatment courses, and little direct data has evaluated the relative efficacy of treatment based on intensity relative to the RMT.

Higher intensities do have significant implications for safety and tolerability. Patient discomfort and pain during treatment and the development of post-treatment headache are certainly more common at higher treatment intensities. In addition, higher intensities are related to a greater risk of seizure induction. The risk of seizure induction is dependent on stimulation intensity, the duration of stimulation trains, and the intertrain interval (see Chap. 14). According to established safety guidelines, when rTMS is applied in high-frequency trains, stimulation can safely be applied up to 120% of the RMT if the stimulation train duration is limited to 4.2 s [10]. Little research has explored the safety implications of the interval between trains: with 10 Hz trains some authors have proposed that the interval should be at least twice the duration of the actual train itself. At lower frequencies, the train can be extended safely to longer durations (see Table 14.1). Note, however, that the safety guidelines have only been established for stimulation in the motor cortex: no equivalent data has been obtained in regard to safety for stimulation in frontal areas used in depression treatment.

Although a specific frequency may be prescribed for a course of treatment, local practice may determine that the intensity be varied depending on factors such as patient tolerability. This may be done in one of two ways: first, the prescribed treatment intensity can be applied and the intensity lowered if this is not tolerated by the patient. Second, the patient may be commenced at a lower treatment intensity during the first treatment session which is then progressively increased depending on tolerability.

In our experience, the latter approach is preferable. If patients experience significant pain at an initial high intensity, they are more likely to be dissuaded from continuing treatment or be hypervigilant during subsequent treatment trains. Hypervigilance may increase scalp muscle contraction, further increasing the unpleasant experience of treatment. In contrast, if a positive experience of treatment is established on a low treatment intensity, intensity may be gradually increased to levels that may not otherwise have been well tolerated. Some idea of the individual patient's tolerance to treatment may be estimated during measurement of the RMT. In more sensitive patients we would recommend commencing treatment around 40% of the RMT and progressively increasing this depending on tolerability. Although it would seem desirable to achieve maximal prescribed intensities (typically 120% of the RMT), brain effects of rTMS are clearly apparent at much lower levels (e.g., 90% of the RMT). It may be preferable to have a patient receive a treatment course at a lower intensity than to drop out of treatment altogether due to lack of tolerability of high-intensity stimulation. This is certainly the case given that the existing clinical data does not strongly suggest a linear relationship between stimulation dose and efficacy.

12.4 Factors Affecting the RMT

As indicated previously, the RMT can be influenced by a number of patient-specific factors such as medication status. Medications that suppress cortical excitability, such as benzodiazepines, are likely to increase the RMT. Importantly, withdrawal of benzodiazepines or withdrawal of other CNS depressant medications such as alcohol is likely to increase cortical excitability and substantially lower the RMT. If patients change CNS active medications or drug use during a course of treatment, the RMT should be reassessed and the intensity of stimulation adjusted if it is considered safe to continue with treatment.

There is also individual variation in the RMT across hemispheres. Although one study found no significant group average differences between left and right RMT in depressed patients [11], for individual patients RMT levels can vary by up to 10% across hemispheres and sometimes even more [12]. Therefore, measurement of the RMT in the hemisphere in which treatment stimulation is to be provided is recommended.

It is also possible that the RMT varies significantly across time even in the absence of changes in external factors such as medication dose. A small number of patients in a 2-week trial of rTMS experienced a significant shift in RMT level that could justify recalibration of treatment dose, although no significant group variation was found [11]. A decision to re-measure the RMT over time should be influenced by considerations as to whether the patient is close to safety thresholds in the baseline dose applied. The baseline RMT level does not appear to influence the outcome of treatment [13].

Note: The intensity of stimulation will vary substantially between different brands of rTMS equipment and between different TMS coil types. If an individual patient is to be treated with more than one device or coil type, it should be established prior to treatment if there is any variation. The easiest way to do this is to measure the resting motor threshold with the different device/coils on several patients to establish the consistency of the measures obtained.

12.5 Clinical Recommendations

Although there are limitations in the applicability of RMT measures to prefrontal areas, at this stage rTMS dosing should be based on individual measurement of the RMT. There are a variety of methods for RMT assessment, a number of which are likely to be equivalent in practical implementation. The most important consideration is that each prescribing clinician is trained in and familiar with the method that he or she is able to apply consistently. The RMT should be assessed at the start of each acute course of treatment to determine dosing based on safety and efficacy considerations in the hemisphere to which stimulation will be applied. It should be reassessed when patients alter their consumption of CNS active drugs. The RMT should also be periodically reassessed when patients have extended treatment courses or maintenance rTMS over time.

References

1. Gomez LJ et al (2020) Conditions for numerically accurate TMS electric field simulation. Brain Stimul 13(1):157–166
2. Gomez LJ, Dannhauer M, Peterchev AV (2021) Fast computational optimization of TMS coil placement for individualized electric field targeting. NeuroImage 228:117696
3. Pridmore S et al (1998) Motor threshold in transcranial magnetic stimulation: a comparison of a neurophysiological method and a visualization of movement method. J ECT 14(1):25–27
4. Hanajima R et al (2007) Comparison of different methods for estimating motor threshold with transcranial magnetic stimulation. Clin Neurophysiol 118(9):2120–2122
5. Westin GG et al (2014) Determination of motor threshold using visual observation overestimates transcranial magnetic stimulation dosage: safety implications. Clin Neurophysiol 125(1):142–147
6. O'Reardon JP et al (2007) Efficacy and safety of transcranial magnetic stimulation in the acute treatment of major depression: a multisite randomized controlled trial. Biol Psychiatry 62(11):1208–1216
7. Qi F, Wu AD, Schweighofer N (2011) Fast estimation of transcranial magnetic stimulation motor threshold. Brain Stimul 4(1):50–57
8. Awiszus F (2011) Fast estimation of transcranial magnetic stimulation motor threshold: is it safe? Brain Stimul 4(1):58–59
9. Gross M et al (2007) Has repetitive transcranial magnetic stimulation (rTMS) treatment for depression improved? A systematic review and meta-analysis comparing the recent vs. the earlier rTMS studies. Acta Psychiatr Scand 116(3):165–173

10. Wassermann EM (1998) Risk and safety of repetitive transcranial magnetic stimulation: report and suggested guidelines from the International Workshop on the Safety of Repetitive Transcranial Magnetic Stimulation, June 5–7, 1996. Electroencephalogr Clin Neurophysiol 108(1):1–16
11. Navarro R et al (2009) Hemispheric asymmetry in resting motor threshold in major depression. J ECT 25(1):39–43
12. Maller JJ et al (2016) Factors to consider when applying transcranial magnetic stimulation of dorsolateral prefrontal cortex when resting motor threshold is asymmetric: a case study. Bioelectromagnetics 37(2):130–135
13. Dolberg OT et al (2002) Magnetic motor threshold and response to TMS in major depressive disorder. Acta Psychiatr Scand 106(3):220–223

Maintenance and Continuation Treatment

13

Abstract

As is the case with other antidepressant therapies, relapse rates appear to be relatively high in the period of time following the cessation of an acute course of rTMS treatment. A number of strategies can be explored to minimize relapse rates. These include the provision of appropriate ongoing antidepressant medication, possibly combined with a mood stabilizer such as lithium. Specific forms of psychotherapy are also likely to have relapse prevention potential although these have not been systematically evaluated following rTMS treatment. A number of methods for the provision of rTMS maintenance have been proposed, although only limited data has explored the efficacy of these to date. These include a "standard" approach of gradually decreasing session intensity and a "clustered maintenance" approach. Patients who have responded well to rTMS treatment and subsequently relapse appear to have a high likelihood of responding to a subsequent course of rTMS treatment with no accumulation of risks or side effects.

13.1 Introduction

To date, in the significant majority of settings in which rTMS has been used in the treatment of depression, it has been applied as a time-limited treatment for a defined depressive episode. However, depression is clearly a relapsing illness and the majority of patients who have responded to rTMS are likely to need some form of treatment to minimize the chances of experiencing relapse and/or maximize the duration of time until this occurs, as is the case with other antidepressant treatments. In the event that relapse occurs, retreatment with rTMS may be a useful option.

P. B. Fitzgerald, Z. J. Daskalakis, *rTMS Treatment for Depression*,
https://doi.org/10.1007/978-3-030-91519-3_13

13.2 Rates of Relapse Following rTMS Treatment

Unfortunately, there appears to be a relatively high relapse rate in the 6–12 months following a successful course of rTMS. This is a situation analogous to that following a successful treatment of depression with ECT, where relapse rates are known to be high and are frequently reported as up to 50% within 6 months [1, 2].

One of the first studies to explore rTMS relapse rates compared relapse rates following successful rTMS or ECT and showed similar rates [3]: 20% of 41 patients in the overall study relapsed over a 6-month period, 4 in each of the ECT and rTMS groups.

One of the largest and most substantive studies of post-rTMS relapse involves the retrospective analysis of the outcomes of 204 patients who had undergone rTMS treatment. All patients had achieved remission of depression with a Hamilton Depression Rating Scale (HAMD) score of less than 8 and were followed for 6 months. Relapse was defined as an increase in HAMD score above 8, a very conservative figure as patients could be defined as having relapsed with only very minor depressive symptoms. Nonetheless, approximately 25% were categorized as having relapsed at 2 months, 40% at 3 months, and 80% by 6 months, obviously a very high figure [4]. An additional study has reported the follow-up of patients who received rTMS treatment in a large multisite trial. Patients who had at least a 25% reduction in HAMD scores during acute rTMS treatment were tapered onto antidepressant medication and followed up over 6 months. Relapse was defined as a recurrence of symptoms sufficient to meet DSM-IV criteria for major depression over 2 consecutive weeks. Ten of 99 (10%) patients relapsed fully over 24 weeks, and a total of 38.4% had substantial symptom deterioration of sufficient severity to justify reintroduction of rTMS treatment (an increase of at least one point on the Clinical Global Improvement—Severity (CGI-S) scale for 2 consecutive weeks) [5]. Fifteen patients experienced a second period of symptom recurrence following an additional course of rTMS, and five patients a third period of symptom recurrence within the 6-month period all justifying further rTMS treatment.

In our clinical experience, and in observation of the patients who have participated in our clinical trials over the last two decades, we have observed that there is a fairly specific pattern of likelihood of relapse. Specifically, there is a subgroup of patients, probably around 20–30%, who will experience a relatively early relapse, within 3 or 4 months of the cessation of their index treatment. There is another group who will achieve sustained and persistent clinical benefit and may not relapse for several years or more. The majority of patients fall somewhere in the middle with relapse likely to occur somewhere between 3 and 24 months after the end of successful treatment. The likelihood of sustained benefit certainly appears to be directly related to the degree of response initially achieved. Patients who have a full resolution of depression are much more likely to have a sustained response than partial responders. These patterns are seen even when patients continue to receive treatment with maintenance antidepressant medication, often in conjunction with additional augmentation agents such as antipsychotics and other mood stabilizers, although patients rarely modify their medication to try to better sustain clinical benefit once they have successfully responded to rTMS (and are much more likely to try and reduce or come off medication).

13.3 Approaches to Minimize Relapse

The first step in minimizing relapse is the identification of those who likely to experience it. Although there has been minimal systematic research in this area, there are likely to be clinical variables that predict the chance of early relapse. For example, and as discussed above, the presence of persistent depressive symptoms despite a significant improvement in overall depression severity is likely to be related to early deterioration once treatment finishes. The presence of substantial ongoing life stressors, marital or work-related conflict, and the presence of substantial axis II or substance-related comorbidity would all seem to be potential predictors of early relapse.

Given the importance of these factors, it is critical to assess each patient toward the end of the course of rTMS treatment for factors that are likely to undermine longer-term outcomes. A direct approach to tackling comorbid issues or social stressors should commence prior to the cessation of active treatment. For example, patients with a history of comorbid substance use problems should be engaged in appropriate therapeutic programs as early as feasible. In the context of ongoing relationship difficulties, family or marital therapy should be considered and potentially commenced prior to the end of rTMS treatment. This will allow issues that are likely to undermine progress to be identified, relevant others to be engaged, and a temporary plan put in place to provide adequate support to the patient while longer-term changes can be undertaken.

Along with the consideration of these factors, an active maintenance plan should be instituted, involving the strategies to be adopted for each individual patient. Maintenance treatment may include antidepressant medication, psychotherapy, and/or further treatment with rTMS.

13.4 Medication Treatment

There is clearly established efficacy for the use of antidepressant medication in the prevention of relapse following initial response to medication. However, little systematic research has investigated whether the recommencement of antidepressant treatment or continuation of antidepressants during and after rTMS treatment will reduce subsequent relapse rates. One study has addressed these issues, although unfortunately only over a very short period of time and in an atypical sample. In this trial, patients with treatment-resistant vascular depression were provided acute treatment with rTMS. After the rTMS course finished, patients were given 20 mg per day of citalopram and evaluated at 3, 6, and 9 weeks. Thirteen of 33 patients responded to rTMS and subsequently received 9 weeks of medication. During this 9-week period four relapsed and nine remained well [6]. In a second study, a small group of patients with bipolar disorder whose depressive episode had responded to rTMS were followed while continuing antidepressant medication [7]. Of six rTMS responders, four remained well over a 12-month period of time. Of the other responders, one relapsed and another partially relapsed after 6 months.

In considering the role of antidepressant medication post-rTMS, some information may be extrapolated from trials of medication treatment post-ECT as this is also a time-limited episodic treatment. Even if patients had previously failed to respond to medication treatment, antidepressant medication may have a role in the prevention of relapse. For example, a small study showed that imipramine substantially reduced post-ECT relapse rates compared to placebo in medication nonresponsive patients [8]. However, antidepressant medication alone may produce suboptimal benefits compared to combination treatment. Sackiem et al. demonstrated that lithium combined with nortriptyline, a tricyclic antidepressant, produced a substantially lower relapse rate and longer time to relapse compared to the antidepressant alone or placebo [9]. A second study has also more recently supported the notion that adding lithium to an antidepressant treatment may reduce relapse post-ECT [10]. In the context of this research, it would be sensible to suggest that where pharmacotherapy is the mainstay of maintenance treatment post-rTMS, a combination of an antidepressant and lithium should be considered. However, although this is a sensible and evidence-based approach, many, if not most, patients are unlikely to be interested in commencing a new medication, especially a complicated one like lithium, soon after they have finally responded to rTMS when medication was not all that helpful for them before. Therefore, this is probably most likely to be a useful strategy in patients who have experienced a relapse already and are looking for an option to try to stay well longer term following a successful second or third course of rTMS.

Of note, no studies have been published exploring the use of new antidepressant agents such as serotonin or serotonin and norepinephrine reuptake inhibitors as maintenance therapy in conjunction with lithium. In general, the choice of medication in this relapse prevention phase is likely to be influenced by factors such as previous tolerance and partial or complete nonresponse to different medication classes. Regardless, in patients who relapse after rTMS with continued antidepressant treatment, the addition of lithium should be strongly considered during subsequent maintenance periods.

13.5 Psychotherapy

An alternative approach to the prevention of relapse post-rTMS treatment is engagement in a form of psychotherapy. Cognitive behavioral therapy (CBT) and its variations are increasingly being utilized in the treatment of depression and in the prevention of depressive relapse. CBT is widely accepted and provided as a first-line treatment for depression, and there are a number of meta-analyses supporting its efficacy (e.g., [11]). Although rates of treatment response to CBT seem to be similar to those achieved with antidepressant medication, CBT appears to have distinct advantages over medication in terms of relapse prevention, with some studies suggesting that patients will relapse at a lower rate after the end of CBT treatment [12–14]. The success of CBT in maintaining treatment benefits has led to it being used as a specific relapse prevention intervention following other acute treatments. Fava et al. [15] used a sequential trial design in which the acute phase of depression was treated with antidepressant medication, with responders then tapered off medication and randomized to receive either a course of CBT or routine clinical management. After 2 years, the patients receiving CBT showed a relapse rate of 25% compared to 80% in the control group. After 6 years the difference was 40% versus 90%, respectively [15]. Another trial found that the combination of CBT with maintenance antidepressant medication following acute episode recovery was superior to maintenance antidepressant medication alone in preventing relapse [16]. This observed advantage persisted several years later [17].

Subsequent trials have refined the delivery of CBT during the maintenance phase by integrating CBT for depression [18] with mindfulness training to create an efficient 8-session course specifically targeting depressive relapse. Mindfulness training is used to develop attention control skills which help the person to more effectively recognize and disengage from patterns of depressive thinking (e.g., hopelessness, guilt, rumination) as they re-emerge, preventing them from escalating. The efficacy of MBCT in minimizing relapse has been established in a series of randomized controlled trials which have found reduced rates of relapse in people with a history of recurrent depression (three or more episodes), compared with routine clinical management alone [19, 20]. A meta-analysis of four of these studies found an average rate of relapse over 12 months of 32% for MBCT compared with 60% for clinical management [21]. A further trial has found that the post-therapy relapse prevention effects of MBCT when antidepressants are withdrawn are at least as effective as continuing maintenance antidepressant medication [22]. Furthermore, there is strong evidence that the relapse-preventing effects of MBCT are mediated by changes in processes targeted by the intervention [23].

Unfortunately, no research to date has assessed the value of CBT or MBCT in the prevention of relapse post-rTMS. One small initial open-label study has explored the role of CBT in the prevention of relapse following ECT [24]. CBT post-ECT was feasible and appeared to enhance duration of persistence of response. However, despite the lack of research, there is no intrinsic reason why these forms of psychotherapy would not be practically useful in the prevention of relapse post-rTMS, and they should be actively considered.

13.6 Maintenance rTMS Treatment

The final possibility is the use of maintenance rTMS to prevent relapse. This has face validity given the response to active treatment in the individual patient. However, maintenance rTMS has only been studied in a limited way to date with limited sham-controlled studies. The most commonly reported maintenance model has been the provision of weekly or fortnightly single rTMS sessions, often with a progressive decrease in session frequency over time. This pattern mimics that which used with maintenance ECT and we will refer to this as the "standard" approach.

13.6.1 Standard Maintenance

The first report of rTMS used for maintenance appeared in 2002 which described a patient who maintained a degree of wellness during 4 months of weekly or twice-weekly rTMS [25]. This was followed by a number of open-label studies and clinical series suggesting the potential benefit of this approach (see reviews in [26, 27]). For example, O'Reardon et al. reported the treatment of ten patients who received maintenance treatment once or twice a week between 6 months and 6 years [28]. They described seven of the patients as having experienced substantial benefit, with three of the seven not requiring medication treatment. In a small open-label follow-up study, Isserles et al. provided weekly dTMS sessions to 11 patients who had remitted to an initial course of dTMS [29]. Ten patients remained in the study and in remission for 4 weeks, while one withdrew due to persistent insomnia. Li et al. reported the maintenance treatment of seven patients with bipolar disorder who were provided with weekly TMS for up to a year [30]. Three patients completed a full year's treatment without substantial relapse.

In a more recent and larger study, 49 patients who had improved with rTMS were randomized to either a single rTMS treatment once per month or no treatment at all [31]. Notably, all patients remained off medication during the study although a further course of rTMS was allowed if patients started to relapse. Patients receiving monthly rTMS sessions had a numerical, but not statistically significant, longer duration until the needed reintroduction of treatment and a numerical but nonsignificant lower rate of treatment reintroduction. It is possible that the failure of the differences in this study to reach significance arose from the limited sample size. It is also notable, however, that just providing a single session once per month may well have been insufficient to maintain substantial wellness.

A second small and undoubtedly underpowered sham-controlled study randomized 17 patients who had responded to TMS to active or sham maintenance provided for 11 months [32]. The schedule reduced from three sessions per week to one session every 2 weeks. There was a greater improvement in depression in the active group in the first 3 months of follow-up, although not after this time when the frequency of rTMS sessions was reduced from weekly to every second week.

A third study included 66 rTMS responders and randomized these to either maintenance rTMS, venlafaxine, or both (note the patients had not previously failed to respond to venlafaxine) [33]. They received 12 months of maintenance beginning twice weekly and then reducing gradually to once every 2 weeks. The percentage of patients who did not meet relapse criteria was similar across three groups, suggesting that rTMS was similar to venlafaxine in the sample.

One additional study that speaks to the potential value of maintenance TMS was conducted using dTMS [34]. A total of 212 depressed subjects who had received either active or sham stimulation over 4 weeks in an initial acute treatment trial then went on to receive two dTMS treatments per week for a further 12 weeks. There was a significant benefit of active over sham stimulation after the initial 4 weeks of treatment (38.4% vs. 21.3% response rate), and this difference remained stable during the 12 weeks of maintenance with a significantly greater number of patients in the active treatment group remaining well at study end (32.6% met response at end vs. 14.6% in the sham group).

13.6.2 Clustered Maintenance

Another possibility is the more intensive provision of multiple sessions, an approach we have termed "clustered maintenance." This essentially involves the application of multiple sessions over a short period of time on a more intermittent basis. We initially commenced this providing five individual treatment sessions over a 3-day period, usually over a weekend, once per month, in patients who have had several depressive episodes successfully treated with rTMS [35]. The "dose" as such was proposed to be similar to that would be received as a once a week. Patients enrolled in this program had experienced a relapse within 3 months at the end of their initial course of rTMS. On response to a second course of rTMS, they were entered into maintenance treatment. In an analysis of 37 patients who were enrolled in this program [35], 21 experienced a relapse after a mean treatment duration of 10.5 months. Six patients continued until study end without relapse (mean of 12 months) and eight withdrew following an average of 6.2 months maintenance treatment without having experienced relapse.

A number of recent studies have also described patients treated using this clustered approach. For example, Pridmore et al. found that some patients returning for this form of intermittent treatment on average demonstrated some degree of early relapse of symptoms (which was generally successfully managed with short burst of treatment sessions) although there was a degree of variability in the duration between treatment applications in this population [36].

The most substantive study in a form of maintenance rTMS published to date investigated the use of clustered maintenance, but in a sample of patients who had responded to medication, rather than rTMS treatment [37]. Two hundred and eight-one patients who had achieved full or partial remission with antidepressant medication were randomized to either rTMS, medication, or combination treatment. Treatment involved ten sessions over a 5-day period monthly for the first 3 months and then five sessions over a 3-day period monthly thereafter. Patients receiving rTMS withdrew from their medication in the first 2 weeks of maintenance treatment.

Overall, there was a significant benefit in both mean time to relapse and total relapse rate for rTMS or combination treatment over antidepressant medication alone. Relapse rates in the rTMS-only group were 24.2%, in the combination group 15.9%, and 44.4% for medication alone. Notably, five patients receiving medication, but none receiving rTMS, experienced a manic switch during the study.

13.7 Other Options: Intermittent Treatment

A final possibility for maintenance rTMS is the use of a targeted intermittent strategy. For example, if a patient has been noted to relapse regularly 6 months post-rTMS, initiating maintenance 5 months after acute treatment and continuing for several months may be a potentially useful approach. Similarly short periods of maintenance treatment could be used every 6 months or so. Alternatively, on demonstration of early signs of relapse, patients could be rapidly re-engaged in a maintenance treatment course of shorter duration. This strategy, however, may not be suitable for a significant proportion of patients who deteriorate rapidly. This sort of approach has not been evaluated systematically in any research that we were aware of.

13.8 Repeated rTMS Treatment

If patients have successfully responded to rTMS treatment and experience a relapse, they are frequently likely to be keen to engage in a further acute course of treatment. Several studies have described populations who have been engaged in retreatment during depressive relapse. The majority of these studies suggest that most patients will successfully respond to treatment when it is applied on a second or subsequent occasion [5, 38, 39]. For example, in a study by Janicak et al., 38 patients were retreated during 24 weeks of follow-up and 32 (84.2%) subsequently improved [5]. We have previously described the treatment of 19 patients over a course of 30 episodes of depressive relapse, where the vast majority of subsequent courses resulted in treatment response [39]. This response pattern has continued into the repeat treatment of now more than 100 patients, some on more than 5 rTMS treatment occasions. However, it is uncommon, and we have noted that a failure to respond to treatment can occur at any subsequent treatment course.

13.9 Summary and Clinical Recommendations

All patients who have responded to a course of rTMS should have an individually developed maintenance relapse prevention treatment plan. For many patients, especially following an initial response to rTMS, this is likely to involve addressing factors that may contribute to relapse, continuing antidepressant treatment, and considering psychotherapy.

Maintenance rTMS may be sensibly considered as an option after an initial clinical response or after relapse and successful retreatment. The decision to use maintenance rTMS, especially after an initial episode of acute treatment, will be influenced by the severity of the initial episode (patients who have been highly disabled by depression may be keen to do anything possible to prevent potential relapse) as well as the availability, suitability, or acceptability of other treatment alternatives such as medication and psychotherapy.

At this stage the research literature does not define the optimal strategy for the initiation of maintenance treatment and one should consider both the standard approach and clustered maintenance. Choice between these two options is likely to be significantly influenced by practical factors such as accessibility and convenience. When using the standard maintenance approach, the evidence suggests that reducing the frequency of treatments to below once every 2 weeks is likely to raise the risk of relapse to an unacceptably high level. However, it would otherwise be sensible to try and reduce the frequency of sessions to the minimum required to maintain wellness for each patient.

References

1. Grunhaus L, Dolberg O, Lustig M (1995) Relapse and recurrence following a course of ECT: reasons for concern and strategies for further investigation. J Psychiatr Res 29(3):165–172
2. Tew JD Jr et al (2007) Relapse during continuation pharmacotherapy after acute response to ECT: a comparison of usual care versus protocolized treatment. Ann Clin Psychiatry 19(1):1–4
3. Dannon PN et al (2002) Three and six-month outcome following courses of either ECT or rTMS in a population of severely depressed individuals—preliminary report. Biol Psychiatry 51(8):687–690
4. Cohen RB, Boggio PS, Fregni F (2009) Risk factors for relapse after remission with repetitive transcranial magnetic stimulation for the treatment of depression. Depress Anxiety 26(7):682–688
5. Janicak PG et al (2010) Durability of clinical benefit with transcranial magnetic stimulation (TMS) in the treatment of pharmacoresistant major depression: assessment of relapse during a 6-month, multisite, open-label study. Brain Stimul 3(4):187–199
6. Robinson RG, Tenev V, Jorge RE (2009) Citalopram for continuation therapy after repetitive transcranial magnetic stimulation in vascular depression. Am J Geriatr Psychiatry 17(8):682–687
7. Dell'Osso B et al (2011) Long-term efficacy after acute augmentative repetitive transcranial magnetic stimulation in bipolar depression: a 1-year follow-up study. J ECT 27(2):141–144
8. van den Broek WW et al (2006) Imipramine is effective in preventing relapse in electroconvulsive therapy-responsive depressed inpatients with prior pharmacotherapy treatment failure: a randomized, placebo-controlled trial. J Clin Psychiatry 67(2):263–268
9. Sackeim HA et al (2001) Continuation pharmacotherapy in the prevention of relapse following electroconvulsive therapy: a randomized controlled trial. JAMA 285(10):1299–1307
10. Rehor G et al (2009) [Relapse rate within 6 months after successful ECT: a naturalistic prospective peer- and self-assessment analysis]. Neuropsychiatrie 23(3):157–163
11. Gloaguen V et al (1998) A meta-analysis of the effects of cognitive therapy in depressed patients. J Affect Disord 49(1):59–72
12. Blackburn IM, Eunson KM, Bishop S (1986) A two-year naturalistic follow-up of depressed patients treated with cognitive therapy, pharmacotherapy and a combination of both. J Affect Disord 10(1):67–75
13. Evans MD et al (1992) Differential relapse following cognitive therapy and pharmacotherapy for depression. Arch Gen Psychiatry 49(10):802–808
14. Simons AD et al (1986) Cognitive therapy and pharmacotherapy for depression. Sustained improvement over one year. Arch Gen Psychiatry 43(1):43–48
15. Fava GA et al (2004) Six-year outcome of cognitive behavior therapy for prevention of recurrent depression. Am J Psychiatry 161(10):1872–1876
16. Paykel ES et al (1999) Prevention of relapse in residual depression by cognitive therapy: a controlled trial. Arch Gen Psychiatry 56(9):829–835

17. Paykel ES et al (2005) Duration of relapse prevention after cognitive therapy in residual depression: follow-up of controlled trial. Psychol Med 35(1):59–68
18. Beck J (1996) Cognitive therapy: basics and beyond. Guilford Press, New York
19. Teasdale JD et al (2000) Prevention of relapse/recurrence in major depression by mindfulness-based cognitive therapy. J Consult Clin Psychol 68(4):615–623
20. Ma SH, Teasdale JD (2004) Mindfulness-based cognitive therapy for depression: replication and exploration of differential relapse prevention effects. J Consult Clin Psychol 72(1):31–40
21. Chiesa A, Serretti A (2011) Mindfulness based cognitive therapy for psychiatric disorders: a systematic review and meta-analysis. Psychiatry Res 187(3):441–453
22. Kuyken W et al (2008) Mindfulness-based cognitive therapy to prevent relapse in recurrent depression. J Consult Clin Psychol 76(6):966–978
23. Kuyken W et al (2010) How does mindfulness-based cognitive therapy work? Behav Res Ther 48(11):1105–1112
24. Fenton L et al (2006) Can cognitive behavioral therapy reduce relapse rates of depression after ECT? A preliminary study. J ECT 22(3):196–198
25. Abraham G, O'Brien S (2002) Repetitive transcranial magnetic stimulation is useful for maintenance treatment. Can J Psychiatry 47(4):386
26. Fitzgerald PB (2019) Is Maintenance Repetitive Transcranial Magnetic Stimulation for Patients With Depression a Valid Therapeutic Strategy? Clin Pharmacol Ther 106(4):723–725.
27. Rachid F (2018) Maintenance repetitive transcranial magnetic stimulation (rTMS) for relapse prevention in with depression: A review. Psychiatry Res 262:363–372.
28. O'Reardon JP et al (2005) Long-term maintenance therapy for major depressive disorder with rTMS. J Clin Psychiatry 66(12):1524–1528
29. Isserles M et al (2011) Cognitive-emotional reactivation during deep transcranial magnetic stimulation over the prefrontal cortex of depressive patients affects antidepressant outcome. J Affect Disord 128(3):235–242
30. Li X et al (2004) Can left prefrontal rTMS be used as a maintenance treatment for bipolar depression? Depress Anxiety 20(2):98–100
31. Philip NS, Dunner DL, Dowd SM, Aaronson ST, Brock DG, Carpenter LL, et al (2016) Can Medication Free, Treatment-Resistant, Depressed Patients Who Initially Respond to TMS Be Maintained Off Medications? A Prospective, 12-Month Multisite Randomized Pilot Study. Brain Stimul 9(2):251–7.
32. Benadhira R et al (2017) A randomized, sham-controlled study of maintenance rTMS for treatment-resistant depression (TRD). Psychiatry Res 258:226–233
33. Haesebaert F et al (2018) Usefulness of repetitive transcranial magnetic stimulation as a maintenance treatment in patients with major depression. World J Biol Psychiatry 19(1):74–78
34. Levkovitz Y et al (2015) Efficacy and safety of deep transcranial magnetic stimulation for major depression: a prospective multicenter randomized controlled trial. World Psychiatry 14(1):64–73
35. Fitzgerald PB, Grace N, Hoy KE, Bailey M, Daskalakis ZJ (2013) An open label trial of clustered maintenance rTMS for patients with refractory depression. Brain Stimul 6(3):292–7.
36. Pridmore S et al (2018) Early relapse (ER) transcranial magnetic stimulation (TMS) in treatment resistant major depression. Brain Stimul 11(5):1098–1102
37. Wang HN et al (2017) Clustered repetitive transcranial magnetic stimulation for the prevention of depressive relapse/recurrence: a randomized controlled trial. Transl Psychiatry 7(12):1292
38. Demirtas-Tatlidede A et al (2008) An open-label, prospective study of repetitive transcranial magnetic stimulation (rTMS) in the long-term treatment of refractory depression: reproducibility and duration of the antidepressant effect in medication-free patients. J Clin Psychiatry 69(6):930–934
39. Fitzgerald PB et al (2006) Naturalistic study of the use of transcranial magnetic stimulation in the treatment of depressive relapse. Aust N Z J Psychiatry 40(9):764–768

14 rTMS Associated Adverse Events, Safety and Monitoring

Abstract

Repetitive transcranial magnetic stimulation is generally considered a safe and well-tolerated interventional tool. However, there are a number of significant contraindications to rTMS stimulation and safety considerations. The major contraindications to rTMS treatment are (1) conditions that substantially predispose an individual to seizure induction, such as history of epilepsy, an active brain illness, or significant alcohol or drug withdrawal, and (2) the presence of programmable devices (such as a pacemaker) or implanted metallic material in the brain that is likely to be adversely affected by strong magnetic fields. The major adverse event concern with rTMS is seizure induction. The likelihood of seizure induction appears to be very low with standard methods of stimulation, and this can be limited by careful patient selection and by closely adhering to established safety guidelines. rTMS stimulation also can induce a syncopal episode, especially in more vulnerable individuals. Fortunately, rTMS does not appear to induce cognitive impairment and there is no evidence of adverse impacts of rTMS stimulation on brain tissue. Hearing protection should be worn during rTMS treatment by patients and treatment providers. Greater care should be taken with the provision of rTMS treatment in special populations such as children or pregnant women.

14.1 Introduction

rTMS treatment is generally very well tolerated. It is notable that the overall discontinuation with rTMS rate is markedly lower than that usually seen in depression treatment trials, especially trials of medication. For example, in the two large multisite rTMS trials, the withdrawal rate in the active groups was 12% and <10% [1, 2]. It is often less than 5% in single site studies (e.g., [3]). It is notable the dropout

P. B. Fitzgerald, Z. J. Daskalakis, *rTMS Treatment for Depression*,
https://doi.org/10.1007/978-3-030-91519-3_14

rates with active rTMS therapy in sham-controlled trials do not appear to be greater in the active treatment groups than in the patient groups receiving the control sham stimulation [4, 5], indicating that treatment emergent adverse events that lead to trimming discontinuation are rare.

Despite the extremely good safety profile of rTMS therapy, there are some clear contraindications to important safety considerations and side effects of rTMS treatment.

14.2 Contraindications

The major contraindications to rTMS treatment fall into two categories:

1. Conditions that raise the risk of seizure induction.

   These conditions include epilepsy or another seizure disorder or other forms of active brain illness such as a recent cerebral vascular accident or a medical condition that substantially raises cortical excitability. In addition, alcohol or drug withdrawal, including withdrawal from benzodiazepines, can substantially increase seizure risk.
2. The presence of material that could interact with the induced magnetic field.

   rTMS may potentially interact with implanted material through the induction of currents (especially in circular wires), through heating, through the induction of movement in magnetically active material, or through changing the parameters of magnetically programmed devices.

An implanted cochlear implant, pacemaker, or other form of magnetically programmable device may be affected by the magnetic field generated with rTMS treatment. Although studies have not investigated the interaction of rTMS with a cochlear implant, these implants contain looped antenna where induced currents are likely to be substantial. rTMS stimulation has been shown outside of the body to induce only small currents in deep brain stimulation electrodes (e.g., [6, 7]). However, only local currents, not currents between the electrode and the pulse generating case, were investigated; these latter currents may be greater. rTMS applied close to the pulse generator can produce substantial damage to the device [6]. Researchers have concluded that rTMS may be safely applied in the presence of other forms of pulse generators (such as vagal nerve stimulation, cardiac pacemakers, and spinal cord stimulators) as long as a substantial distance is maintained between the implanted wires/pulse generator and where the TMS coil is discharged [8]. Padding (such as a lifejacket) may be put in place to prevent accidental stimulation close to the pulse generator [9]. We have safely administered rTMS therapy in patients with pacemakers in situ but have taken a number of precautions while doing so. One practical thing that we have implemented has been to make sure that the patient is as fully reclined as possible and their head tilted slightly backward. This places the TMS coil in a position such that if there was a failure of the coil stand, the coil would slip backward over the head and onto the floor rather than down toward the chest where there would be a greater risk of the coil coming into closer contact with the pacemaker itself.

rTMS could also potentially interact with medically implanted metal components in the skull or brain. Skull plates are most commonly made from titanium which is non-ferromagnetic and has low conductivity, lessening the likelihood of significant interaction [10]. However, if a titanium plate was in the region of the frontal cortex, it could certainly distort the magnetic field being received by the targeted area of the brain and as such one would be more inclined to stimulate on the opposite side, away from this metal. Aneurysm clips are frequently cited as a contraindication to rTMS treatment, though one study has calculated that the energy imparted on aneurysm clips would move these minimally in a manner unlikely to produce clinical problems [11].

A further area of relative contraindication to rTMS treatment is the presence of medical problems that could be destabilized if a seizure induced by rTMS was to occur. For example, the presence of substantial ischemic cardiac disease could be a concern as a patient may not have the necessary cardiac reserve to tolerate the physiological stresses associated with a seizure. However, the potential benefit of rTMS treatment needs to be weighed against this concern, especially as the risk of seizure is quite low.

14.3 Adverse Events

14.3.1 Syncope

The major safety concern with rTMS treatment has been related to the potential for seizure induction (see below). However, syncope ("fainting") is another mechanism through which patients may lose consciousness during a medical procedure such as rTMS, and it is possible that this occurs more commonly than seizure. Syncopal reactions are relatively common following medical procedures such as blood taking, and there appears to be a group of individuals susceptible to this type of reaction.

Syncopal reactions are brief and have no long-term consequences. However, it can be difficult to distinguish these from rTMS-induced seizures. This diagnostic problem arises if patients display behavioral manifestations while unconscious that might be attributed to seizure activity. Seizure-like activity, including muscle jerks and tonic muscle activity, can occur during syncopal episodes. However, tongue biting or incontinence is infrequent during syncopal episodes and is more likely to indicate seizure activity. Syncopal episodes are frequently preceded by a patient experiencing light-headedness, a need to lie down, nausea, and a sensation of heat. Notably, patients will recover consciousness fully within seconds, in a much more rapid manner than would be expected following a seizure, where full consciousness may take several minutes to re-establish. There is no definitive test to permit the delineation of these two types of episodes: prolactin may be elevated following a generalized seizure but does not have adequate specificity to be relied on clinically.

The immediate management of a patient who has lost consciousness during TMS does not depend on whether the diagnosis of syncope or seizure is made at the time. Regardless, the patient should be assisted to lie in a prone position on one side and the airway protected as required. Movement of the subject undergoing a tonic clonic seizure should not occur until motor activity has ceased. Evaluation following the event is likely to involve neurological review, including the possibility of the conduct of an EEG.

14.3.2 Seizure Induction

The major risk with rTMS treatment is the induction of seizure activity [12, 13]. A number of seizures were reported with TMS prior to the delineation of safety guidelines defining safe stimulation parameters [13]. Since that time, rTMS use has expanded rapidly and large numbers of subjects have undergone stimulation protocols across a variety of psychiatric and neurological disorders. Despite this marked increase in use, there have only been sporadic published reports of seizure induction and mainly in conditions other than depression. All of the reported seizures occur with rTMS treatment during or immediately after stimulation trains. There is no evidence that rTMS produces changes in brain activity that predispose individuals to experience seizures some time following the end of stimulation. In addition, where seizures have occurred, there is no evidence that individuals have developed a propensity to experience seizures in the future, or have experienced ongoing adverse consequences.

Box 14.1 Stimulation Parameters and Seizure Risk

The likelihood of seizure induction is related to several aspects of stimulation characteristics: stimulation frequency, train duration, intensity, and the duration of time between rTMS trains. Safety guidelines have been published describing what are known to be safe combinations of these parameters. For example, when stimulation is applied at 10 Hz, 5 s is considered a safe train duration when stimulation is applied at up to 110% of the resting motor threshold (Table 14.1). This train duration is reduced to 4.2 s at 120% of the RMT and 2.9 s 130% of the RMT. It should be noted that the vast majority of research that has informed these guidelines has been conducted with stimulation of the primary motor cortex. It is not clear whether the same guidelines should directly translate to other non-motor brain areas. However, providing stimulation in experimental and treatment studies within these guidelines has not resulted in a substantial rate of seizures. Therefore, in the absence of alternative data, these guidelines should be followed unless a clear rationale is provided, and informed consent obtained with an awareness of the novelty of stimulation parameters.

Table 14.1 Established safe stimulation parameters for individual trains (adapted from [8])

	Intensity (% of the RMT)				
Frequency	90	100	110	120	130
1	>1800	>1800	<1800	>360	>50
5	>10	>10	>10	>10	>10
10	>5	>5	>5	4.2	2.9
20	2.05	2.05	1.6	1.0	0.55
25	1.28	1.28	0.84	0.4	0.24

The maximum established safe train duration for motor cortical stimulation based on varying frequencies and intensities. Stimulation in excess of the safe train duration may result in the development of seizures or seizure-like brain activity. Durations marked with a ">" are the maximal tested durations

A number of the seizures reported since the publication of safety guidelines in 1998 [13] have occurred when stimulation was provided outside of safety guidelines. For example, a generalized seizure was reported following stimulation with 10 Hz trains of 10-s duration in a patient with chronic pain (at 100% of the RMT) [14]. A second generalized seizure occurred in a patient with major depression during 15 Hz stimulation provided via 10-s trains at 110% of the RMT [15]. The majority of seizures reported using deep TMS to Brainsway since clinical approval of deep TMS for depression have been when the treatment system has been used outside of recommended guidelines [16]. In fact, only 14 seizures out of 55 that were reported between 2010 and 2020 occurred when the use instructions were followed.

There have clearly been, however, seizures reported where stimulation was provided within the 1998 and later safety guideline. For example, in one patient with bipolar disorder, a generalized seizure was induced during single pulse TMS measurement of the RMT [17]. Notably, this patient had a family history of epilepsy and was concurrently taking chlorpromazine and lithium. A second seizure was reported during RMT assessment, but this time in a patient with multiple sclerosis [18]. A generalized seizure was reported in a patient with tinnitus receiving rTMS treatment at 1 Hz [19], although the possibility that this was syncopal has been raised [20]. A single seizure has also been reported using continuous theta-burst stimulation, an experimental paradigm involving repeated application of three train pulses at 50 Hz [21].

There have been several attempts to try to quantify seizure risk from published reports although these are universally challenged by the lack of consistent publicly available information. Lerner et al. surveyed laboratories and clinics to obtain information on TMS sessions and seizure induction between 2012 and 2016 [22]. Twenty-four seizures were reported during the conduct of 318,560 experimental and clinical TMS sessions for a rate of 0.08 per 1000 sessions. When just considering TMS delivered within safety guidelines to patients without significant risk factors, they only identified 4 seizures for a risk of about 1 seizure every 60,000 sessions.

More recently Chou et al. conducted a literature search investigating rates of seizure reports up until February 2020 [23]. They found 41 reports of seizures, 13 healthy individuals in experimental paradigms, and 28 in patients with psychiatric or neurological conditions. Fifteen seizures were reported in patients with mood or anxiety disorders and a total of only 34% (14 seizures) were reported with prefrontal stimulation.

The most systematic data and seizure frequency has been collected for the Brainsway deep TMS system [16]. A total of 55 seizures were reported between 2010 and 2020 from a total of 94,857 patients treated during that time. This provides a seizure frequency of 6 per 10,000 patients although the rate of seizure induction when treatment was provided following the use guidelines was only to pretend 1000 patients. Interestingly, and with potential clinical relevance, the report described the possibility that significant voluntary movements during rTMS could have been associated with six of the seizures that occurred when treatment was provided following the clinical use guidelines. It is possible that voluntary movement, by increasing excitability of the motor cortex and potentially the prefrontal cortex, could play a significant role in increasing risk.

It is notable that even in patients with a substantial risk for seizure induction, rTMS-related seizures are rare. A review of the safety of rTMS in patients with epilepsy found that less than 2% of patients experienced an event during rTMS (4 of 280 patients) [24].

Monitoring of EEG during rTMS treatment does not appear to provide information likely to be useful in the prevention of seizure induction. As evident in a review [8], multiple studies have explored the induction of transient epileptiform activity during rTMS treatment. This is occasionally detectable in patient groups, but does not appear to be of use in monitoring treatment [8].

A number of conditions increase the risk of seizure induction necessitating avoidance of the rTMS procedure or use with considerable caution. The most widely identified risk factor is the presence of a past history of a seizure disorder, especially epilepsy. This is considered an absolute contraindication to a course of rTMS in most circumstances although we have reported the successful treatment of a patient with a history of epilepsy with low-frequency right-sided treatment [25]. Some programs have historically excluded patients with a family history of epilepsy but we are not aware of any reported cases of seizures induced in individuals who fall into this group.

Beyond epilepsy, there are a range of neurological conditions which are likely to increase risk of seizures, most likely when there is an active pathophysiological process underway [26]. However, TMS treatment has been successfully applied in clinical trials and a range of conditions including Parkinson's disease, post-stroke, post-traumatic brain injury, and Alzheimer's disease without reports of significant rates of seizure induction. However, significant caution should be taken if there is the presence of an active brain condition when considering recommendations for rTMS therapy.

It is also worthy of note that the presence of unstable cardiac disease also requires caution due to the increased demands that could be placed on the cardiovascular system in the event of a seizure.

There are a range of pharmacological substances that are likely to alter the seizure threshold and place patients at a somewhat higher risk of seizure induction but for which there is no direct evidence of a significant real-world risk that would leave these to be considered an absolute contraindication. In the analysis of Lerner et al., only three seizures were reported in patients who were suspected of taking medications that could alter the seizure threshold [22]. These would include drugs such as clozapine and bupropion. The treatment of patients on these medications would seem reasonable when otherwise clinically justified but may warrant care being taken to reduce or minimize any other potential causes of increased risk, for example, avoiding treatment during sleep deprivation [26].

What is likely to be of more significance is changes in drug dose that occur between the time when a patient undergoes a resting motor threshold (RMT) assessment and then has treatment or which occurs during the course of treatment. Significant changes in medication dose, especially when the medication is one that may affect seizure threshold, such as a benzodiazepine or anticonvulsant, should result in a recheck of the RMT and adjustment of stimulation dose as appropriate. Significant medication withdrawal would fall into this category. For example, benzodiazepine withdrawal is associated with the spontaneous onset of seizures and would pose a particularly high risk of rTMS-induced seizure activity.

Illicit drug withdrawal, especially from alcohol, would also substantially raise the risk of seizure occurrence. Persistent alcohol misuse, including of a binge nature, should be considered at least a relative contraindication to rTMS therapy.

Finally, there is an association between sleep deprivation and increase seizure risk and so monitoring of sleep patterns during a course of treatment is a sensible precaution.

Note there are ways to at least partially mitigate the risks described to allow treatment to progress in a patient where clinically warranted. For example, seizure induction is likely to be related to stimulation intensity, and a more modest dose, for example, 110% of the RMT, in patients at higher risk of seizure may be warranted (see Box 14.1). Another option is the use of low-frequency stimulation applied to the right DLPFC. Seizure risk does appear to be related to stimulation frequency and as such low-frequency stimulation is likely to propose a much lower risk in vulnerable patients.

14.4 Other Potential Safety Concerns

14.4.1 Impairment of Cognition

The potential for rTMS treatment to produce cognitive impairment has been a concern since the initial development of the procedure. Given the cognitive side effects that complicate the use of ECT, it is a reasonable concern. Clearly, if rTMS is able to produce lasting brain changes sufficient to ameliorate depressive symptoms, it could potentially also produce brain changes with negative implications. Indeed, transient disruption of cognition is a well-recognized effect of stimulation at certain brain sites (e.g., [27]), though enhanced function is reported in other domains [28, 29, 30].

The main question, therefore, is whether deleterious effects of rTMS on cognition persist after stimulation or develop with repeated applications of rTMS during a treatment course. Fortunately, neither appears to be the case. A range of studies have investigated cognitive function in patients with depression, before and after a course of rTMS. For example, in an early study, Little et al. tested 16 cognitive measures after 1 week of 1 Hz and 1 week of 20 Hz rTMS at 80% of the RMT in a crossover design and reported no adverse effects. No deterioration in cognitive function was also reported in an open study of 2 weeks of 20 Hz rTMS administered at 80% of the RMT [38]. Loo et al. analyzed cognitive outcomes across 39 clinical studies [12]. Although in three studies deterioration on one or more cognitive tests was reported, a substantially greater number of studies reported cognitive improvement, and no specific pattern of cognitive deterioration was apparent across the trials. An analysis of potential cognitive side effects of rTMS was also included in the pivotal Neuronetics Ltd.-sponsored clinical trial [3]. In this study up to 216,000 pulses were applied to patients, typically 3000 pulses per day over an hour, each day, for 6–9 weeks at 120% of the RMT. No cognitive deterioration was noted across the Mini-Mental State Examination, the Autobiographical Memory Interview, or the Buschke Selective Reminding Test.

It is notable that cognitive improvement seen in rTMS studies in depression in other contexts has led to an increased interest in research in the use of rTMS as a tool to actually improve cognition. This has led to trials in a variety of disorders including Alzheimer's disease (e.g., [31, 32]), suggesting at a minimum that rTMS is able to produce short-term improvements in cognition. This literature would seem to provide additional reassurance that rTMS generally speaking is likely to be a cognitively safe intervention.

The conclusion that is most appropriately drawn from these studies is that there is no current evidence that rTMS as applied in its standard clinical forms for the treatment of depression produces cognitive side effects. However, as rTMS dosing and modes of application change over time, especially with the development of increasingly high-dose protocols, cognitive safety will require continued reappraisal. The potential capacity of rTMS to produce enduring changes in brain function should also be considered when rTMS is being used in an off-label manner.

14.4.2 Hearing Impairment

When an rTMS machine produces its magnetic field, a substantial sound is generated by the deformation of the stimulating coil. At times this sound may exceed what is considered to be safe for direct exposure to the ear, with sound levels of up to 140 dB [33]. In early studies, some changes in auditory thresholds were reported in individuals exposed to rTMS stimulation, although these reports were not of permanent changes (e.g., [34]). A persistent decrease in auditory thresholds was reported in a patient stimulated with a deep TMS (H-coil) who was not using hearing protection during the procedure [35]. A series of more recent studies have reported no changes in hearing thresholds, when rTMS is provided with appropriate hearing protection (e.g., [2]). Hearing safety of rTMS in children has not been fully established [8].

It is recommended that hearing safety is optimized by the use of well-fitted hearing protection with earplugs or earmuffs in patients undergoing rTMS treatment as well as for rTMS operators [26]. It is also recommended that treatment only be applied with considerable caution in patients undergoing treatment with ototoxic medication such as aminoglycosides or cisplatin.

14.4.3 Potential Histotoxicity or Other Brain Changes

It is possible that rTMS stimulation could produce damage to brain tissue either through heating effects, through effects mediated through the produced magnetic field, or to the effects of the induced electrical fields. In regard to the former, heating effects induced by TMS stimulation appear to be minimal and are likely to be limited by the dissemination of heat through natural brain perfusion. There are no known mechanisms through which the induced magnetic field produced during TMS stimulation could generate biological adverse effects in the absence of extraneous implanted metal in the skull or brain. Magnetic forces on ferromagnetic objects such as metallic brain implants could produce displacement of these objects. Skull plates are most commonly titanium which is non-ferromagnetic. One report has shown minimal heating of titanium skull plates with 1 Hz rTMS [10].

Studies of the effects of the induced electrical fields on brain tissue take a number of approaches. Animal studies using direct electrical stimulation have produced pathological changes in brain tissue, but only after extensive periods of stimulation at charge levels markedly in excess of that induced with rTMS stimulation [36]. Animal experiments investigating more standard TMS stimulation have failed to clearly demonstrate evidence of induced pathological changes. However, the interpretation of these studies is considerably confounded by inequities in the application of rTMS across animal and human situations [12]. One animal study reported microvacuolar changes with stimulation intensities equivalent to three times motor threshold, but this finding has not been replicated in at least four other studies that have shown no adverse changes (for review see [37]).

Studies have also looked at the potential effects of rTMS on various brain parameters in human subjects. These have shown no adverse effects on the blood-brain barrier [38], no changes in gross brain structure (with MRI) [39], and no adverse effects on EEG, ECG, and neurohormonal levels [40]. One human pathological study revealed no adverse changes in the brains of two patients with epilepsy who underwent rTMS prior to surgery [41].

A further consideration is whether exposure to the magnetic field generated during rTMS has potential adverse consequences. This is especially relevant considering the ongoing debate regarding potential health and safety concerns with exposure to pulsed electromagnetic field (EMF) from mobile phones and other sources. Given the average duration of the TMS magnetic pulse and the number of pulses in treatment courses, it has been calculated that the typical treatment course would provide exposure of only short duration (e.g., 5 s) [12]. Presumably this would increase with higher doses and longer courses of rTMS as are now currently being evaluated. However, exposure duration would still remain very short compared to other sources of EMF. The nature of the exposure also varies significantly from other sources: TMS-related exposure has high intensity and is pulsed for brief duration, compared to the low intensity, but continuous exposure is potentially related to other devices. The implications of this variation are unclear, but to date there has been no evidence of any safety-related concerns or complications arising in regard to EMF exposure and rTMS treatment. Although it is typically assumed there are no direct brain effects of the magnetic field produced during TMS other than those of the secondary electrical field, it is possible that this is not the case. Neurones do contain material that is potentially magnetically manipulable [42]. However, the implications of this manipulation potential to the actions of rTMS remain completely unknown.

14.5 Pregnancy, Breastfeeding

As discussed in Chap. 5, the use of rTMS in pregnancy has only been described in a limited number of case series (e.g., [43]) and small clinical trials. No adverse events or negative fetal outcomes have been documented to date which have been able to be attributed to rTMS therapy. Modeling of the electrical field produced by TMS stimulation also suggests that there is no exposure of risk to the fetus [44, 45]. Twenty-six children born to mothers who received TMS treatment during pregnancy were followed up for up to 62 months with no evidence of any significant perinatal complications or abnormalities in cognitive or motor development [46]. However, the accumulated number of patients treated to date is clearly inadequate to make firm conclusions about safety. There is also the theoretical possibility that the sound produced by the rTMS coil could have some deleterious effect on the developing hearing of the fetus. The consent of patients for treatment who are pregnant should reflect this in addition to other risk-benefit-associated issues.

A similar conclusion can be made about the use of rTMS in the treatment of patients who are postpartum and breastfeeding. Although rTMS treatment could potentially induce changes in hormonal secretion and breast milk composition, there is no evidence of this or associated harmful effects. In addition, hormonal fluctuations associated with breastfeeding may change cortical excitability, elevating the risk of seizure induction. These risks are likely to be small.

14.6 Children and Adolescents

Data collected on the use of rTMS in children and adolescents has been extremely limited to date, although large numbers of subjects under 18 have participated in single pulse and paired pulse experimental protocols. One seizure in a 16-year-old female patient has been reported with relatively low-dose stimulation parameters. This could indicate the possibility of a higher rate of seizure induction in this population, given that the total number of adolescent patients reported as having received treatment in the literature is very low. However, making inferences from a single case is significantly problematic. A study in 2017 reviewed published data from more than 200 studies applying TMS in experimental and clinical context to about 2000 children finding no evidence of significant safety concerns [47]. Adolescent patients may also be at a higher risk of experiencing syncopal episodes.

14.7 Safety of Operators

As rTMS becomes increasingly utilized in clinical practice, the safety of operators is likely to become the focus of increasing concern. To date, it is not an area to which substantial consideration has been addressed. One study has explored the exposure of staff applying rTMS to magnetic fields, comparing measured and extrapolated fields to European safety guidelines [48]. The authors propose that staff should maintain a distance of at least of 0.7 m from the coil while treatment is underway. However, testing was conducted with only one rTMS device, at a limited range of stimulation parameters. A more recent study has also evaluated the field exposure with the same magnetic simulator (MagPro with MC-B70 figure-of-eight coil) and concluded that the distance required to minimize exposure to that below the safety limit was 40 cm.

A recent study has used full-body field modeling to investigate the fetal exposure in a potentially pregnant TMS operator. This analysis suggested that a distance of greater than 60 cm was required to minimize exposure below the specific risk levels defined in the International Commission on Non-Ionizing Radiation Protection (2003, 2017) [44].

Given that all rTMS treatment coils currently available can be held in place with a holding arm system, it seems sensible to ensure that these are always used when treatment is underway. The operator of the rTMS equipment can then be standing or seated at least 1 m from the coil during treatment, except when making brief checks of coil positioning. We would also recommend that staff administering rTMS wear appropriate ear protection due to the prolonged and repeated exposure to rTMS-related noise.

References

1. George MS et al (2010) Daily left prefrontal transcranial magnetic stimulation therapy for major depressive disorder: a sham-controlled randomized trial. Arch Gen Psychiatry 67(5):507–516
2. O'Reardon JP et al (2007) Efficacy and safety of transcranial magnetic stimulation in the acute treatment of major depression: a multisite randomized controlled trial. Biol Psychiatry 62(11):1208–1216
3. Janicak PG et al (2008) Transcranial magnetic stimulation in the treatment of major depressive disorder: a comprehensive summary of safety experience from acute exposure, extended exposure, and during reintroduction treatment. J Clin Psychiatry 69(2):222–232

4. Berlim MT et al (2014) Response, remission and drop-out rates following high-frequency repetitive transcranial magnetic stimulation (rTMS) for treating major depression: a systematic review and meta-analysis of randomized, double-blind and sham-controlled trials. Psychol Med 44(2):225–239
5. Zis P et al (2020) Safety, tolerability, and nocebo phenomena during transcranial magnetic stimulation: a systematic review and meta-analysis of placebo-controlled clinical trials. Neuromodulation 23(3):291–300
6. Kumar R, Chen R, Ashby P (1999) Safety of transcranial magnetic stimulation in patients with implanted deep brain stimulators. Mov Disord 14(1):157–158
7. Kofler M, Leis AA (1998) Safety of transcranial magnetic stimulation in patients with implanted electronic equipment. Electroencephalogr Clin Neurophysiol 107(3):223–225
8. Rossi S et al (2009) Safety, ethical considerations, and application guidelines for the use of transcranial magnetic stimulation in clinical practice and research. Clin Neurophysiol 120(12):2008–2039
9. Schrader LM et al (2005) A lack of effect from transcranial magnetic stimulation (TMS) on the vagus nerve stimulator (VNS). Clin Neurophysiol 116(10):2501–2504
10. Rotenberg A et al (2007) Minimal heating of titanium skull plates during 1Hz repetitive transcranial magnetic stimulation. Clin Neurophysiol 118(11):2536–2538
11. Barker AT (1991) An introduction to the basic principles of magnetic nerve stimulation. J Clin Neurophysiol 8(1):26–37
12. Loo CK, McFarquhar TF, Mitchell PB (2008) A review of the safety of repetitive transcranial magnetic stimulation as a clinical treatment for depression. Int J Neuropsychopharmacol 11(1):131–147
13. Wassermann EM (1998) Risk and safety of repetitive transcranial magnetic stimulation: report and suggested guidelines from the International Workshop on the Safety of Repetitive Transcranial Magnetic Stimulation, June 5–7, 1996. Electroencephalogr Clin Neurophysiol 108(1):1–16
14. Rosa MA et al (2006) Accidental seizure with repetitive transcranial magnetic stimulation. J ECT 22(4):265–266
15. Prikryl R, Kucerova H (2005) Occurrence of epileptic paroxysm during repetitive transcranial magnetic stimulation treatment. J Psychopharmacol 19(3):313
16. Tendler A et al (2021) Seizures provoked by H-coils from 2010 to 2020. Brain Stimul 14(1):66–68
17. Tharayil BS et al (2005) Seizure with single-pulse transcranial magnetic stimulation in a 35-year-old otherwise-healthy patient with bipolar disorder. J ECT 21(3):188–189
18. Haupts MR et al (2004) Transcranial magnetic stimulation as a provocation for epileptic seizures in multiple sclerosis. Mult Scler 10(4):475–476
19. Nowak DA et al (2006) Epileptic seizure following 1 Hz repetitive transcranial magnetic stimulation. Clin Neurophysiol 117(7):1631–1633
20. Epstein CM (2006) Seizure or convulsive syncope during 1-Hz rTMS? Clin Neurophysiol 117(11):2566–2567. author reply 2567–2568
21. Oberman L, Pascual-Leone A (2009) Report of seizure induced by continuous theta burst stimulation. Brain Stimul 2(4):246–247
22. Lerner AJ, Wassermann EM, Tamir DI (2019) Seizures from transcranial magnetic stimulation 2012–2016: results of a survey of active laboratories and clinics. Clin Neurophysiol 130(8):1409–1416
23. Chou YH et al (2020) TMS-induced seizure cases stratified by population, stimulation protocol, and stimulation site: a systematic literature search. Clin Neurophysiol 131(5):1019–1020
24. Bae EH et al (2007) Safety and tolerability of repetitive transcranial magnetic stimulation in patients with epilepsy: a review of the literature. Epilepsy Behav 10(4):521–528
25. Fitzgerald PB (2014) Treatment of depression in a patient with epilepsy. Brain Stimul 7(4):619–620
26. Rossi S et al (2021) Safety and recommendations for TMS use in healthy subjects and patient populations, with updates on training, ethical and regulatory issues: expert guidelines. Clin Neurophysiol 132(1):269–306

27. Jahanshahi M, Ridding MC, Limousin P, Profice P, Fogel W, Dressler D et al (1997) Rapid rate transcranial magnetic stimulation–a safety study. Electroencephalogr Clin Neurophysiol 105(6):422–429
28. Wassermann EM, Grafman J, Berry C, Hollnagel C, Wild K, Clark K et al (1996) Use and safety of a new repetitive transcranial magnetic stimulator. Electroencephalogr Clin Neurophysiol 101(5):412–417
29. Foltys H, Sparing R, Boroojerdi B, Krings T, Meister IG, Mottaghy FM, Töpper R (2001) Motor Clin Neurophysiol 112(2):265–274
30. Boroojerdi B, Phipps M, Kopylev L, Wharton CM, Cohen LG, Grafman J (2001) Enhancing analogic reasoning with rTMS over the left prefrontal cortex. Neurology 56(4):526–528
31. Chou YH, Ton That V, Sundman M (2020) A systematic review and meta-analysis of rTMS effects on cognitive enhancement in mild cognitive impairment and Alzheimer's disease. Neurobiol Aging 86:1–10
32. Velioglu HA et al (2021) Left lateral parietal rTMS improves cognition and modulates resting brain connectivity in patients with Alzheimer's disease: possible role of BDNF and oxidative stress. Neurobiol Learn Mem 180:107410
33. Counter SA, Borg E (1992) Analysis of the coil generated impulse noise in extracranial magnetic stimulation. Electroencephalogr Clin Neurophysiol 85(4):280–288
34. Loo C et al (2001) Effects of a 2- to 4-week course of repetitive transcranial magnetic stimulation (rTMS) on neuropsychologic functioning, electroencephalogram, and auditory threshold in depressed patients. Biol Psychiatry 49(7):615–623
35. Zangen A et al (2005) Transcranial magnetic stimulation of deep brain regions: evidence for efficacy of the H-coil. Clin Neurophysiol 116(4):775–779
36. McCreery DB et al (1990) Charge density and charge per phase as cofactors in neural injury induced by electrical stimulation. IEEE Trans Biomed Eng 37(10):996–1001
37. Lorberbaum JP, Wassermann E (2000) Safety concerns of TMS. In: George MS, Belmaker RH (eds) Transcranial magnetic stimulation in neuropsychiatry. American Psychiatric Press, Washington, DC, pp 141–162
38. Niehaus L et al (2000) MRI study of human brain exposed to high-dose repetitive magnetic stimulation of visual cortex. Neurology 54(1):256–258
39. Nahas Z et al (2000) Lack of significant changes on magnetic resonance scans before and after 2-weeks of daily left prefrontal repetitive transcranial magnetic stimulation for depression. J ECT 16(4):380–390
40. Pascual-Leone A et al (1993) Safety of rapid-rate transcranial magnetic stimulation in normal volunteers. Electroencephalogr Clin Neurophysiol 89(2):120–130
41. Gates JR, Dhuna A, Pascual-Leone A (1992) Lack of pathologic changes in human temporal lobes after transcranial magnetic stimulation. Epilepsia 33(3):504–508
42. Dobson J (2002) Investigation of age-related variations in biogenic magnetite levels in the human hippocampus. Exp Brain Res 144(1):122–126
43. Nahas Z et al (1999) Safety and feasibility of repetitive transcranial magnetic stimulation in the treatment of anxious depression in pregnancy: a case report. J Clin Psychiatry 60(1):50–52
44. Yanamadala J et al (2019) Estimates of peak electric fields induced by transcranial magnetic stimulation in pregnant women as patients or operators using an FEM full-body model. In: Makarov S, Horner M, Noetscher G (eds) Brain and human body modeling: computational human modeling at EMBC 2018. Springer, Cham, pp 49–73
45. Yanamadala J et al (2017) Estimates of peak electric fields induced by transcranial magnetic stimulation in pregnant women as patients using an FEM full-body model. Annu Int Conf IEEE Eng Med Biol Soc 2017:1441–1444
46. Kim DR et al (2019) Randomized controlled trial of transcranial magnetic stimulation in pregnant women with major depressive disorder. Brain Stimul 12(1):96–102
47. Allen CH, Kluger BM, Buard I (2017) Safety of transcranial magnetic stimulation in children: a systematic review of the literature. Pediatr Neurol 68:3–17
48. Karlstrom EF et al (2006) Therapeutic staff exposure to magnetic field pulses during TMS/rTMS treatments. Bioelectromagnetics 27(2):156–158

Side Effects of rTMS Treatment

15

Abstract

Absolutely, and compared to other antidepressant treatments, rTMS is generally well tolerated. The most common side effects experienced by patients are pain or discomfort at the site of stimulation and the development of a headache. These side effects may be moderated by the method of the application of stimulation although in a very small percentage of subjects, treatment will remain intolerable. It is possible that rTMS treatment in depressed subjects can induce mania although reports of this have predominately been in patients with bipolar disorder. If the field of stimulation overlaps with the motor cortex, muscle twitching in the contralateral limb can be observed and care needs to be taken to distinguish these from muscle twitching-associated epileptiform discharges.

15.1 Introduction

rTMS is generally very well tolerated, as best illustrated by the very low dropout rates seen in clinical trials which have been shown to be equivalent to that seen in groups of patients receiving sham stimulation [1]. The most commonly reported side effects of rTMS treatment are the occurrence of discomfort or pain during stimulation, and the development of a headache during or after treatment. Inductions of psychiatric symptoms, muscle tension, or seizure are also possible.

15.2 Site or Regional Pain

Discomfort at the site of stimulation or headache is the most common side effect seen in patients undergoing TMS treatment reported in almost 20% of patients in placebo-controlled studies compared to about 10% in the sham groups [1].

P. B. Fitzgerald, Z. J. Daskalakis, *rTMS Treatment for Depression*,
https://doi.org/10.1007/978-3-030-91519-3_15

Treatment-related discomfort or pain is usually experienced directly beneath the TMS coil. However, it can also be experienced in the forehead, the region of the upper eyelid, or even an upper jaw tooth. Pain is most likely to relate to trigeminal nerve stimulation and direct muscle contraction. It is also possible that head fixation during treatment sessions will produce pain through neck discomfort.

The experience of discomfort or pain is highly variable between individuals; it may be strongly influenced by coil location or orientation as well as the intensity and frequency of stimulation. Despite this relatively high rate symptoms seen in clinical trials, discontinuation due to discomfort is infrequent and does not seem to differ from that seen with sham stimulation [1].

A variety of methods have been explored to reduce treatment-related discomfort. Researchers have used topical or locally injected anesthetic agents or inserted air-filled or foam pads between the coil and the scalp surface. A substantial beneficial effect was seen with local anesthetic injection but not with the other techniques in a pilot study [2]. The commercially available Neuronetics Ltd.-manufactured rTMS device has a single use disposable attachment designed to reduce local discomfort. However, no systematic studies have been published exploring whether this attachment has clinical benefit.

Stimulation-related discomfort may be reduced in several practical ways (see Box 15.1). First, small modifications of coil position or orientation may lessen the sensation produced with stimulation. Given the inherent inaccuracy with standard methods of coil localization, although it has not been systematically assessed, there is no reason to believe that small coil modifications would substantially affect treatment efficacy. Second, a decrease in stimulation intensity will reduce discomfort in most patients. Given that there seems to be a relationship between stimulation intensity and efficacy, this decrease should be limited. However, antidepressant effects of rTMS have been seen from 90% to 120% of the RMT and may well still be produced if intensity is decreased from the higher stimulation levels.

Box 15.1 Practical Strategies to Minimize Scalp Discomfort and Pain

- Shift coil 0.5–1.0 cm toward the midline.
- Shift coil 0.5–1.0 cm posterior.
- Rotate handle of coil ~20° toward the midline.
- Reduce stimulation intensity.
- Switch to low-frequency stimulation.

Anxiety also appears to be a factor determining the intensity of rTMS-related discomfort. Therefore, in most patients it is sensible to begin treatment at a low stimulation intensity that is likely be tolerable to allow patients to become comfortable with the sensation. Stimulation intensity can then be progressively increased over the first treatment week [3] (see Box 15.2). In our experience this is a more sensible approach than starting stimulation at full intensity and reducing if required.

This later approach may establish a strong negative expectation and association with treatment that may be long-lasting. It is important to note that discomfort may well lessen over several treatment sessions with consistently applied intensity [4, 5]. In one study, a substantial reduction in pain occurred in the first few days with a steady progressive reduction continuing throughout 3 weeks of treatment [5].

Box 15.2 Commencing Treatment to Maximize Tolerability
We recommend that the first rTMS treatment session be commenced at an intensity significantly under the planned treatment intensity to maximize the likelihood that patients will tolerate their overall course of treatment. We would typically commence stimulation at around 40% of the RMT and gradually increased this over the course of one or more treatment sessions depending on individual patient tolerability. A slower commencement of higher intensity stimulation is likely to enable the patient to relax more during treatment, reducing the likelihood of voluntary scalp muscle contraction and contributing to stimulation-related discomfort.

When treatment remains intolerable with the strategies explored above, a switch from high-frequency left-sided 10 Hz stimulation to low-frequency right-sided rTMS is a worthwhile consideration. Low-frequency stimulation is generally better tolerated than its high-frequency counterpart [6] and 1 Hz stimulation can often be tolerated at extremely high intensities.

15.3 Headache

Headache is the other common side effect experienced with rTMS treatment. It has been reported in about 28% of patients provided active treatment compared to 16% with sham across clinical trials [7]. Headache can be reported during stimulation or afterward treatment. On occasion this does require the use of analgesic medication; some patients may benefit from taking these before their treatment sessions commence.

15.4 Other Transient Side Effects

A range of side effects have been reported in clinical trials but not at rates greater than sham stimulation typically (see Box 15.3). Dizziness can occur with TMS although relatively uncommonly: ~3% of patients compared to 2% of patients with sham stimulation [1] but this difference was not statistically significant.

Box 15.3 Reported Side Effects from rTMS Treatment

- Application site discomfort or pain
- Headache
- Eye or facial pain
- Muscle twitching
- Toothache
- Nausea
- Dizziness
- Insomnia
- Fatigue
- Anxiety
- Back/neck pain

These are side effects reported in some of the large randomized controlled trials. Rates of most of these do not differ between active and sham stimulation group.

15.5 Psychiatric Complications

The major potential psychiatric complication of rTMS treatment for patients with mood disorders is the induction of mania. This has been documented across a number of case studies (e.g., [8–10]), which include treatment with rTMS in patients with bipolar disorder. Some researchers suggested that switch rates may not substantially be greater than with sham treatment compared to left-sided rTMS, low-frequency right-sided rTMS, and bilateral stimulation. Manic induction has been reported predominately in patients with bipolar disorder, but also in several patients with unipolar depression [10, 11]. Xia et al. in 2008 summarized the early literature on manic induction finding only 13 cases across over 50 randomized trials [12]. The reported rates of manic switch with active treatment were only marginally greater than that seen with sham rTMS (0.84% vs. 0.73%) and low compared to what would be expected without treatment. This suggests rTMS may not elevate manic switch rates. Whatever the relationship between rTMS treatment and mania induction, it seems sensible to warn patients undergoing treatment of this possibility, particularly those with bipolar disorder. It would be reasonable to advise patients who have experienced substantial manic episodes in the past, especially episodes compromising their wellbeing, to take a mood stabilizer during their course of rTMS treatment.

In one case reported by George et al. [11], manic symptoms resolved when treatment scheduling was reduced from daily to every second day. We have had similar experiences with several patients who have been able to be successfully treated by reducing the intensity of treatment scheduling, despite early emerging manic symptoms. We have also seen some patients with an increase in what might be considered "sub-manic symptoms" such as insomnia, agitation, or anxiety [13] which have been able to be moderated by reducing session frequency.

A second, but less well-validated, concern is the potential induction of psychotic symptoms during rTMS treatment. The development of persecutory delusions was reported in a single case study of a non-psychotically depressed subject. In this instance, a causative relationship was suggested due to a close temporal relationship with treatment [14], and the possibility that it resulted from subcortical dopamine release has been raised. Regardless, if the induction of psychotic symptoms is related to rTMS treatment, it seems a highly infrequent possibility given the large numbers of rTMS patients who have undergone treatment in recent years without further reports.

Overall, rates of psychiatric side effects have not differed between active and sham groups in large clinical trials conducted to date [13].

15.6 Other Considerations

There are no other side effects consistently reported in randomized trials as occurring at greater frequency with active stimulation compared to sham [1]. Muscle twitching was reported in 20% of the subjects in the Neuronetics Ltd.-sponsored pivotal trial, but it was not specified whether this occurred only during stimulation or whether it was a persistent effect post-treatment [15]. Muscle twitching in the contralateral arm during rTMS treatment can occur through the inadvertent placement of one wing of a figure-of-eight coil close enough to the motor cortex to cause neuronal depolarization in this brain region. When muscle twitching occurs during rTMS treatment, it is important to try and differentiate whether it is arising through direct stimulation of the motor cortex, or whether it could be occurring via spreading neuronal excitation from prefrontal to motor areas. The latter may be the precursor of a seizure event.

With direct motor cortex stimulation, twitching will occur during the stimulation train and cease immediately at the end of the train. Twitching should also be substantially reduced in magnitude or cease altogether with forward movement or rotation of the coil such that the posterior wing is less adjacent to the motor cortex. Motor cortical stimulation due to spreading excitation will result in muscle twitching that persists beyond the end of the stimulation train. If this is noted to occur, treatment should cease until review. At a minimum, review should entail re-measurement of the motor threshold to ensure that the subject is not being treated at excessively suprathreshold intensity. If spreading excitation is noted at standard stimulation doses following re-measurement of the RMT, strong consideration should be given to stopping rTMS and looking at other treatment alternatives.

References

1. Zis P et al (2020) Safety, tolerability, and nocebo phenomena during transcranial magnetic stimulation: a systematic review and meta-analysis of placebo-controlled clinical trials. Neuromodulation 23(3):291–300
2. Borckardt JJ et al (2006) Reducing pain and unpleasantness during repetitive transcranial magnetic stimulation. J ECT 22(4):259–264
3. Perera T et al (2016) The clinical TMS society consensus review and treatment recommendations for TMS therapy for major depressive disorder. Brain Stimul 9(3):336–346
4. Janicak PG et al (2008) Transcranial magnetic stimulation in the treatment of major depressive disorder: a comprehensive summary of safety experience from acute exposure, extended exposure, and during reintroduction treatment. J Clin Psychiatry 69(2):222–232
5. Anderson BS et al (2009) Decreasing procedural pain over time of left prefrontal rTMS for depression: initial results from the open-label phase of a multi-site trial (OPT-TMS). Brain Stimul 2(2):88–92
6. Kaur M et al (2019) Low-frequency rTMS is better tolerated than high-frequency rTMS in healthy people: empirical evidence from a single session study. J Psychiatr Res 113:79–82
7. Loo CK, McFarquhar TF, Mitchell PB (2008) A review of the safety of repetitive transcranial magnetic stimulation as a clinical treatment for depression. Int J Neuropsychopharmacol 11(1):131–147
8. Ella R et al (2002) Switch to mania after slow rTMS of the right prefrontal cortex. J Clin Psychiatry 63(3):249
9. Hausmann A et al (2004) Can bilateral prefrontal repetitive transcranial magnetic stimulation (rTMS) induce mania? A case report. J Clin Psychiatry 65(11):1575–1576
10. Sakkas P et al (2003) Induction of mania by rTMS: report of two cases. Eur Psychiatry 18(4):196–198
11. George MS et al (1995) Daily repetitive transcranial magnetic stimulation (rTMS) improves mood in depression. Neuroreport 6:1853–1856
12. Xia G et al (2008) Treatment-emergent mania in unipolar and bipolar depression: focus on repetitive transcranial magnetic stimulation. Int J Neuropsychopharmacol 11(1):119–130
13. Rossi S et al (2021) Safety and recommendations for TMS use in healthy subjects and patient populations, with updates on training, ethical and regulatory issues: expert guidelines. Clin Neurophysiol 132(1):269–306
14. Zwanzger P et al (2002) Occurrence of delusions during repetitive transcranial magnetic stimulation (rTMS) in major depression. Biol Psychiatry 51(7):602–603
15. O'Reardon JP et al (2007) Efficacy and safety of transcranial magnetic stimulation in the acute treatment of major depression: a multisite randomized controlled trial. Biol Psychiatry 62(11):1208–1216

The Use of rTMS in Other Psychiatric Disorders

16

Abstract

rTMS treatment is clearly most well established for depressive disorders. However, a considerable body of research has investigated its use in other clinical areas. The second established application for the use of TMS treatment that is now increasingly being utilized in clinical practice is the use of deep TMS in the treatment of obsessive-compulsive disorder (OCD). In schizophrenia, evidence does not consistently show an effect on general positive symptoms. However, there is a suggestion that prefrontal rTMS may modulate negative symptoms and cognition and substantive evidence that left temporoparietal stimulation can reduce the intensity and frequency of auditory hallucinations. There is inconsistent evidence, with many studies not replicated, supporting the use of rTMS in mania or anxiety disorders. There is emerging evidence to suggest that rTMS may modulate the experience of pain although studies are required to better establish its therapeutic use from a longer-term perspective in patients with chronic pain syndromes.

16.1 Introduction

As has been described in previous chapters, rTMS can have powerful effects on the brain. These effects can be neurophysiological (e.g., altering inhibition and plasticity), clinical (e.g., improvement of symptoms in patients with treatment-resistant depression), and cognitive (i.e., transient cognitive lesions, cognitive enhancement). As well as the development of rTMS methods for depression, in the last two decades there has been significant investigation into the treatment of numerous other psychiatric and neurological disorders. While a comprehensive review of all of these findings is beyond the scope of this chapter, we will focus on psychiatric disorders and

P. B. Fitzgerald, Z. J. Daskalakis, *rTMS Treatment for Depression*,
https://doi.org/10.1007/978-3-030-91519-3_16

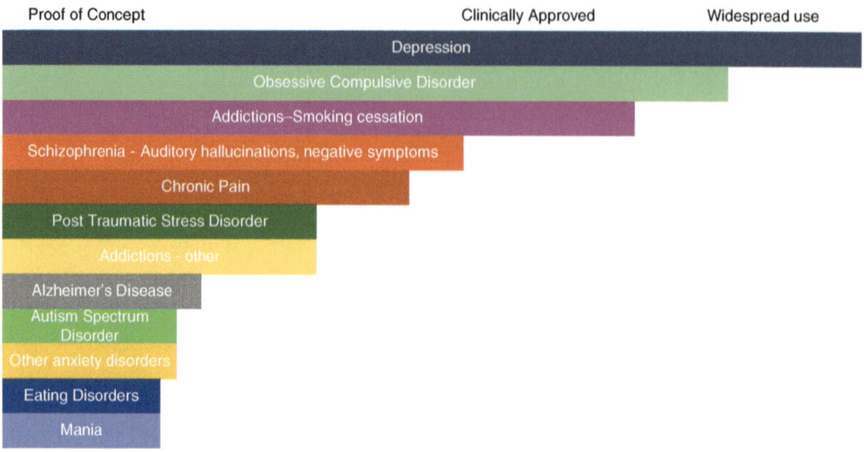

Fig. 16.1 A representation of the clinical development status of rTMS in multiple disorders. Please note clinical approval status does vary substantially across jurisdictions

the greatest evidence that exists for the clinical utility of rTMS approaches or in which there has been particular therapeutic interest (see Fig. 16.1).

16.2 Obsessive-Compulsive Disorder (OCD)

There is a compelling argument for evaluating the use of rTMS in obsessive-compulsive disorder (OCD). OCD can be highly disabling and patients with OCD often respond poorly to psychotherapy and/or serotonergic antidepressants, the standard forms of treatment. Moreover, unlike MDD which responds well to ECT, there is little to no evidence for therapeutic improvement of OCD with ECT. There is also a compelling mechanistic link between treatment mechanisms linked to rTMS and those mechanisms that are aberrant in OCD. For example, rTMS has been reported to potentiate GABAergic neurotransmission, particularly at high frequencies [1, 2]. rTMS can also modulate NMDA neurotransmitter mechanism [3], both of which have been associated with dysfunction in OCD [4, 5]. As such, not only is there is an urgent need for newer treatments in OCD but rTMS may target putative mechanisms in the cortex that are associated with OCD pathophysiology.

Greenberg et al. initially explored the efficacy of rTMS for OCD [6]. Twelve patients received 20 Hz rTMS at 80% of the motor threshold to the right or left lateral prefrontal cortex or a control site. Right prefrontal stimulation decreased compulsions and improved mood to a greater degree than left-sided stimulation or control site stimulation. Several studies that have subsequently explored high-frequency stimulation applied to the left DLPFC have reported mixed results [7, 8]. Several studies have also explored low-frequency approaches to stimulation of the dorsal prefrontal cortex, again, with mixed effects. For example, Alonso et al. reported the effects of 1 Hz rTMS applied to the right DLPFC over eighteen 20 min daily sessions [9]. There were no significant effects on obsessions or compulsions reported. Prasko et al. also used 1 Hz stimulation but applied to the left DLPFC and failed to find therapeutic effects [10]; a second study of 3 weeks of daily right-sided 1 Hz stimulation reported positive effects [11].

Promising results have also been achieved with stimulation of targets outside the DLPFC as would likely be predicted from an understanding of the neuroimaging data underpinning our understanding of the pathophysiology of OCD. The first of these novel approaches was targeting of the bilateral supplementary motor area. An open study and a second controlled study, conducted by Mantovani et al., have suggested the possible therapeutic value of 1 Hz rTMS applied bilaterally to this site [12, 13]. The supplementary motor area is strongly connected to the anterior cingulate, a cortical region that was previously reported to be closely associated with the pathophysiology of OCD [13]. However, one subsequent study combining both 1 Hz stimulation of the right DLPFC and 1 Hz stimulation of the supplementary motor area failed to find positive results [14]. A series of more recent studies, both open-label and double-blind, have presented mixed results (e.g., [15–17]).

A second novel approach has been the application of low-frequency stimulation to the left or right orbitofrontal cortex [18, 19], an approach that appears to offer some potential clinical benefits but which needs to be established in larger-scale clinical trials.

The most significant development in the application of TMS treatment in OCD has been the conduct of trials establishing the effectiveness of deep TMS. Carni et al. published a multicenter randomized double-blind trial of high-frequency (20 Hz) deep TMS targeting the medial prefrontal cortex and anterior cingulate cortex in 99 patients with persistent OCD [20]. The protocol involved a process of symptom provocation immediately prior to the application of deep TMS treatment. Active treatment resulted in a 38% response rate compared to 11% in the sham group with persistent benefits at 1-month follow-up. A subsequent study exploring real-world outcomes and several hundred patients using this protocol has reported quite substantial clinical response rates [21].

Studies exploring the use of various forms of TMS in OCD have been summarized in several recent meta-analysis. For example, a study by Perera et al. included a total of 26 studies with 781 participants [22]. Overall there was a modest reduction in OCD symptom severity across studies with the largest effect sizes obtained with bilateral DLPFC stimulation. Liang et al. found evidence for therapeutic effects of low- or high-frequency stimulation of DLPFC and for low-frequency stimulation of the supplementary motor area [23]. The evidence from these studies, however, clearly indicates that forms of rTMS other than deep TMS require evaluation in larger multisite clinical trials.

16.2.1 Summary

Interpreting the results of studies that have explored the clinical benefits of TMS treatment in OCD is significantly complicated by the diversity of treatment targets utilized in different treatment studies. There is relatively inconsistent evidence from a variety of relatively small studies of potential benefit of treating OCD with stimulation to the DLPFC, supplementary motor area, and orbitofrontal cortex. There is more substantial data from a multisite randomized controlled trial and a second study reporting outcomes in real-world clinical practice, supporting the use of deep TMS applied to dorsomedial prefrontal regions, combined with a provocation protocol. This has led to the FDA approval in the USA of the use of both the H7 Brainsway coil and a double cone coil produced by MagVenture.

16.3 Mania

Due to the promising therapeutic effects of rTMS in depression, interest in the use of the treatment for mania developed early. In an initial study, 16 patients were randomized in a controlled trial of right versus left high-frequency (20 Hz) prefrontal stimulation [24]. Greater therapeutic benefits were seen with right-sided compared to left-sided stimulation, an observation that has been subsequently used to support notions of left- and right-sided laterality activity differences in depression and mania. The therapeutic possibilities with high-frequency right-sided stimulation were also supported in two subsequent case series [25, 26].

However, data from sham-controlled trials is not consistent. In the first of these studies involving 25 patients, no difference between active and sham stimulation was seen [27]. However, in a more recent study of 41 patients, a significant benefit of active over sham 20 Hz stimulation was seen with stimulation over a 10-day period [28].

16.3.1 Summary

A limited body of research suggests that high-frequency stimulation applied to the right DLPFC may have some anti-manic effects but this treatment needs to be more systematically evaluated.

16.4 Post-traumatic Stress Disorder

A series of mostly single site studies have explored the potential application of rTMS in post-traumatic stress disorder (PTSD). The first of these explored the application of very low-frequency stimulation (0.3 Hz) applied to both the left and right motor cortex, producing a reduction in PTSD symptoms [29]. However, this was an uncontrolled study. Subsequently, studies have investigated a variety of stimulation paradigms including low- and high-frequency stimulation applied to the left DLPFC and low- and high-frequency stimulation applied to the right DLPFC [30–33]. High-frequency right-sided stimulation has shown promise in several studies which have evaluated stimulation to both hemispheres or compared different frequencies of stimulation applied to the right DLPFC [31, 32]. Given that neuroimaging-based models of PTSD have suggested that hypoactivity of the DLPFC is associated with hyperactivity of the amygdala and underlying illness symptoms, and that right-sided changes are predominant in PTSD, a high-frequency approach to right-sided stimulation has some therapeutic rationale [34].

Several approaches have been taken to combine rTMS stimulation with some form of psychological treatment or symptom provocation. One approach combined pre-symptom provocation and deep TMS of the medial prefrontal cortex reporting significant therapeutic benefits [35]. The therapeutic benefit was seen when rTMS was applied immediately after exposure to a trauma-related event script. A more recent study reported an approach which combined a weekly session of rTMS and 12–15 weeks of cognitive processing therapy [36]. The group who received combined treatment improved to a greater degree than in patients who received therapy and sham stimulation.

A recent meta-analysis of rTMS studies in PTSD identified 11 randomized controlled trials [37]. Promisingly, the authors found that rTMS produced a significant reduction in core PTSD symptoms with a large effect size and that significant effects were seen with both high- and low-frequency stimulation of the right DLPFC. These effects were seen to be durable at 2 and 4 weeks post-cessation of treatment.

16.4.1 Summary

rTMS appears to have significant potential in the treatment of PTSD. Although the optimal treatment parameters have yet to be confirmed, there seems to be growing evidence for the potential value of low-frequency stimulation applied to the right DLPFC.

16.5 Panic Disorder and Generalized Anxiety Disorder

Following several case reports, two randomized controlled trials have explored the use of rTMS in panic disorder, both investigating 1 Hz stimulation applied to the right DLPFC. In the first study, no significant difference was seen between active and sham stimulation in 15 medication-resistant patients [38]. The second study, in a slightly larger sample size ($n = 25$), did find significant differences in response between active and sham stimulation [39].

Few studies have explored the possible use of rTMS in generalized anxiety disorder (GAD). The first was an open-label study where 1 Hz stimulation was applied to the right DLPFC with the site determined by an fMRI activation scan [40]. Six out of ten patients met remission criteria for reduction in anxiety symptoms within this study. A significant benefit of active over sham stimulation was seen in a small randomized controlled trial of 1 Hz stimulation applied to the right DLPFC [41]. Of note, improvements in anxiety symptoms are commonly seen when depression is treated in patients with anxiety comorbidity, and these improvements and anxiety have been noted with right, left, and bilateral forms of rTMS [42]. No studies have explored the use of rTMS in social anxiety disorder other than case reports [43, 44].

16.5.1 Summary

Only limited research has explored the application of rTMS in panic disorder and GAD. There appears to be a possibility of therapeutic value of 1 Hz stimulation applied to the right DLPFC but at this stage this has very limited empirical support.

16.6 Schizophrenia

Despite some advances in pharmacotherapy over the last 20 years, a significant percentage of patients with schizophrenia experience disabling refractory symptoms. Furthermore, side effects are common with current pharmacotherapy for schizophrenia resulting in high rates of early treatment discontinuation [45]. Thus, researchers and clinicians have sought novel treatments to target refractory symptoms. rTMS has been relatively extensively investigated as a treatment for schizophrenia vis-à-vis positive (e.g., hallucinations and delusions) and negative symptoms of schizophrenia, as well as cognitive dysfunction.

Increasingly schizophrenia researchers consider this disorder to be highly heterogeneous. Therefore, it follows that specific treatment of individual subcomponents of the syndrome, such as the negative symptoms or hallucinations, may yield greater success than nonspecific treatments applied to all patients. It is unlikely that a brain stimulation technique that targets one brain region would likely to improve multiple dimensions of the illness, but may have specific value in ameliorating particular symptoms.

In this regard, rTMS protocols for treatment-resistant schizophrenia have targeted two main cortical areas with differing aims. Dysfunction in the prefrontal cortex is thought to underlie some of the positive and negative symptoms in schizophrenia. Initial treatment protocols targeting the dorsolateral prefrontal cortex (DLPFC) in schizophrenia were inspired by treatment protocols used for major depression. Analogous to the situation in depression, hypoactivation in prefrontal regions is thought to correlate with negative symptoms [46]. Thus, it was hypothesized that high-frequency rTMS applied to the DLPFC may improve negative symptoms by increasing cortical activity [47]. The other main cortical region targeted in rTMS studies has been the temporoparietal cortex (TPC). Although there are some contradictory findings, a number of studies have suggested that the pathophysiology of auditory hallucinations is related to hyperactivity in the left TPC [48, 49]. Based on this understanding, Hoffman et al. developed a low-frequency rTMS protocol applied to the left TPC to modulate the overactive state underpinning auditory hallucinations [50, 51].

16.6.1 Prefrontal Stimulation in Schizophrenia

Early rTMS studies in schizophrenia targeted the DLPFC for a nonspecific treatment. The first published study used only 30 single rTMS pulses applied openly in a single treatment session and described some short-lived therapeutic effects [52]. In a second small open study, a statistically significant decrease in Brief Psychiatric Rating Scale (BPRS) scores was observed after ten sessions of 1 Hz stimulations applied to the right DLPFC [53]. The improvement was primarily seen in nonspecific symptoms, such as anxiety and tension, rather than in the core symptoms of schizophrenia. A larger, controlled study with similar stimulation parameters failed to confirm any significant improvement in schizophrenia symptoms when rTMS was compared to a sham control [54].

High-frequency stimulation to the DLPFC as a treatment for positive symptoms was first studied in a small crossover design comparing left-sided active vs. sham stimulation [55]. A significant reduction in BPRS scores was seen with active but not with sham stimulation. However, three other studies of high-frequency stimulation of the left DLPFC have failed to demonstrate an improvement in positive symptoms [56–58]. A recent meta-analysis concluded that high-frequency stimulation of the DLPFC has failed to show improvement in positive symptoms as assessed by the positive and negative syndrome scale-positive (PANSS-P) or the scale for the assessment of positive symptoms (SAPS) [59].

16.6.2 Negative Symptoms

In contrast to the negative results found when targeting positive symptoms with high-frequency rTMS to the DLPFC, the treatment of negative symptoms with this approach has yielded somewhat more encouraging results. There have been a series of small parallel design trials. In several studies, there were no differences between active and sham groups [56, 60, 61]. However, a series of studies have shown a significant advantage of active over sham stimulation (e.g., [58, 62–64]). Of note, three of these studies [58, 62, 63] used higher stimulation intensity (>100% of the standard resting motor threshold), and one of the studies used a longer treatment duration (15 days) than the negative studies (10 days) [62]. One of these two positive studies also carefully controlled for the possible confound of improved depressive symptoms using scores on the Calgary Depression Scale for Schizophrenia as a covariate: improved depression did not account for the observed improvement in negative symptoms [58]. Another study compared 20 Hz stimulation to stimulation provided at the patient's individual α-frequency with a sham condition [65]. α-frequency stimulation was calculated as the patient's peak α-frequency from five frontal EEG leads. The rationale for enhancing activation by using the patient's own α-frequency was based on the hypothesis that a deficiency in oscillation at this frequency is related to the underlying pathophysiology of negative symptoms.

Stimulation at the patient's α-frequency resulted in a significantly greater reduction in negative symptoms than the other three conditions. Two studies investigating the use of bilateral high-frequency stimulation have both reported no improvement in negative symptoms [66, 67].

A number of larger studies have attempted to confirm whether rTMS may have benefit in the treatment of negative symptoms. For example, Wobrock et al. randomized 175 patients to receive either active (10 Hz rTMS applied to the left DLPC) or sham stimulation for 3 weeks [68]. No statistically significant differences were seen between active or sham treatment at the end of treatment or during subsequent follow-up. However, Quan et al. randomized 117 patients to a longer 20-day course of left prefrontal 10 Hz stimulation (this actually consisted of two 10-day periods of treatment separated by a break of 2 weeks) [69]. The overall dose of stimulation was quite low (800 pulses per day applied at only 80% of the motor threshold) and stimulation applied with a circular coil. It is not clear from the report how the coil was orientated and whether this would have resulted in any bilateral stimulation. A significant benefit of active over sham treatment was seen at 2 weeks and 6 weeks, for negative but not positive symptoms. A third smaller, much smaller, multicenter trial randomized 32 patients to active or sham treatment, provided again at 10 Hz, but this time bilaterally over 3 weeks [70]. A significant difference between active and sham treatment was found for negative but not positive symptoms which persisted at 3-month follow-up.

Finally, a study was recently reported that compared the application of three forms of rTMS applied to the left-sided DLPFC (10 Hz, 20 Hz, and iTBS) to a sham group [71]. All three active groups produced better outcomes in regard to negative symptoms than the control group. The TBS condition produced greater effects than the 10 and 20 Hz rTMS approaches.

Meta-analyses summarizing the results of studies using TMS in the treatment of negative symptoms have generally reported positive results (e.g., [72, 73]) and acknowledged the short-term duration of the treatment trials and effects reported.

16.6.3 Cognition

Only a very small literature has presented studies investigating the effect of rTMS applied to the DLPFC on cognition in patients with schizophrenia. Impaired cognition has been increasingly recognized as a primary deficit in schizophrenia [74]. Recent data suggests that high-frequency rTMS applied to DLPFC can improve performance on higher-order cognitive functions and selectively modulate γ oscillations in frontal regions [75]. Given the prominence of cognitive deficits in patients with schizophrenia, and the potential relationship of aspects of cognition such as working memory to high-frequency EEG oscillations, it seems worthwhile to investigate the effect of high-frequency rTMS of the DLPFC on cognition. Initially, all Barr et al. reported that bilateral rTMS applied at 20 Hz and targeted to the DLPFC could improve working memory deficits in schizophrenia in a study including 27 patients [76]. Working memory was assessed using the N-back task. rTMS significantly improved three-back accuracy to targets compared to sham. There was also a trend toward significance on the effects of rTMS on the one-back versus three-back accuracy, suggesting that rTMS was more effective on working memory performance as difficulty increased.

Subsequent to this, a number of small studies have explored the effects of high-frequency stimulation (typically 10 or 20 Hz) on cognitive variables with mixed results [71, 77, 78]. A recent meta-analysis of 9 studies including 351 patients reported that TMS treatment resulted in improved working memory but not therapeutic benefits on other cognitive domains [79].

16.6.4 Summary

There is relatively consistent evidence to suggest that rTMS may improve negative symptoms of schizophrenia, and possibly some cognitive domains, but these effects have only been reported in the short term from trials conducted over limited periods of time. It is not yet clear how well these effects are likely to translate into clinical practice.

16.6.5 Temporoparietal Cortex rTMS and Auditory Hallucination

The most extensively investigated application for rTMS in schizophrenia has been the use of low-frequency stimulation applied to the left TPC (see Fig. 16.2), in an effort to ameliorate auditory hallucinations (AH). Initial studies were of a relatively short duration but they still demonstrated a decrease in the frequency and intensity of AH [50, 51]. A larger, controlled study, of 9 days of low-frequency left-sided (LFL) stimulation of the TPC found a substantial and significant reduction in AH compared to sham. Furthermore, this improvement was sustained in more than half of the improved subjects at 15 weeks post-treatment [80]. In an even larger controlled study, the efficacy finding was confirmed and the treatment demonstrated an excellent safety and tolerability profile (a consistent finding across subsequent studies) [81].

Several investigators have attempted to replicate and extend these findings using open, crossover, and parallel randomized controlled designs with mixed results [82–93]. Of note, however, is an open study that correlated response to treatment with reduction in cortical metabolism (as measured by PET imaging) beneath the site of stimulation, substantiating the theoretical rationale for this treatment [90]. The mixed results likely relate to heterogeneity in the duration and intensity of treatment. Interestingly, two of the randomized controlled studies have found significant reduction in frequency and intensity of AH with less than 10 days of treatment [82, 83].

An initial meta-analysis of all acute rTMS treatment studies of AH found an effect size of 0.76 (95% CI = 0.36–1.17) for LFL rTMS applied to the left TPC, despite variation in the duration and methods of stimulation [94]. More recent

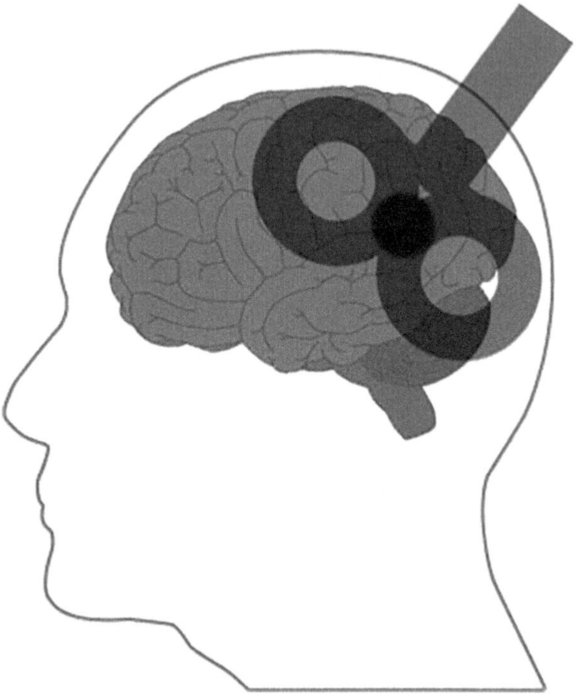

Fig. 16.2 The localization of the TMS coil over temporoparietal junction

meta-analyses have confirmed the finding of a medium to large effect size for therapeutic benefits [95–99]. However, these studies have identified the need for better follow-up and the need for studies of maintenance treatment in patients that respond to an acute course of rTMS.

In an attempt to optimize efficacy, investigators have also started to explore bilateral and right-sided TPC stimulation. Another approach taken to optimizing efficacy has been the utilization of MRI and fMRI to more specifically target the neuroanatomical structures involved in auditory hallucinations. The first study found no specific benefit of rTMS or of MRI-based localization [100]. A second study found an overall benefit with rTMS, but again, no improvement with fMRI-based localization [101]. In another study, LFL rTMS was applied to a series of sites activated on fMRI scan for eight intermittent hallucinators or to a series of sites functionally coupled to Wernicke's area in eight patients with continual hallucinations [102]. Stimulation at the left TPC site resulted in a greater rate of reduction in auditory hallucination severity compared to stimulation at other sites. A novel imaging and treatment protocol in a case report has recently been published [103]. The investigators identified the area of highest activation during a language task using fMRI. The area is correlated with the left superior temporal gyrus. They theorized that high-frequency stimulation (20 Hz) may reduce AH based on work showing disruption in higher cognitive functions such as speech production [104]. A follow-up study with rTMS targeted to the site identified on individual fMRI scans, in a group of 11 patients, demonstrated decreased global severity and frequency of AH in 8 of 11 patients, with a large effect size after only 2 days (2600 pulses) of treatment [105]. This is a striking finding that warrants further investigation with a randomized controlled study. The improvement was present 10 days after treatment in the whole sample and sustained for a mean of approximately 2 months. However, the cost of fMRI localization may be prohibitive for application to the wider population of patients experiencing refractory AH. Therefore, refinements in defining an optimal TPC site that can be found by approximation are necessary.

Beyond some follow-up data provided in a minority of studies, there is minimal data on the longer-term implications of treating AH with rTMS [81]. Fitzgerald et al. reported the successful retreatment of two patients who had relapsed following successful rTMS treatment, one of them on two occasions [106]. There is a report of maintenance rTMS in a patient for 6 months with some decrease in severity but no delay in relapse [107] and a second case where maintenance treatment was successful over an 8-month period [108]. One further case report described a patient who experienced improvement in AH after 1 week of treatment (twice-daily low-frequency stimulation to the left TPC) and also in the second occasion following relapse 6 months later. After the relapse, the patient had sustained improvement over 1 year with once monthly treatment [109]. We have treated a number of patients with repeated courses of rTMS for relapse of hallucinations and achieved consistent responses over time. We have also successfully utilized a clustered maintenance schedule (five treatment sessions over 3 days every 4 weeks) in a small sample of patients with particularly difficult to treat symptoms and frequent relapse.

16.6.6 Summary

A reasonably substantial research base has indicated that low-frequency rTMS applied to the left temporoparietal cortex appears to have therapeutic benefits in ameliorating auditory hallucinations. Given the often very disabling nature of these symptoms, clinical use of this technique could be justified in certain cases although overall response rates may not be high.

16.7 Disorders of Addiction

Disorders of addiction or substance dependence have attracted considerable interest as potential targets for rTMS treatment although much of the research in this area has been conducted with single session studies investigating the capacity of stimulation to modulate intermediate effects such as craving rather than overall clinical outcomes. TMS treatment in addiction has predominately involved applying high-frequency stimulation to the DLPFC to either moderate craving or inhibitory control [110]. Studies have investigated the effects of TMS on a diverse range of addictions including those related to alcohol, opiates, cocaine, and cannabis [110].

The most meaningful clinical progress has been with exploring the use of rTMS in aiding smoking cessation. A series of small clinical trials have demonstrated potential benefits with standard forms of rTMS, and these benefits have been seen in early studies of deep TMS at high but not low frequency [111].

In a recent follow-up to this, the manufacturer of deep TMS coils, Brainsway, has completed a pivotal study of deep TMS in smoking cessation that has been used in a successful FDA application for licensing in the USA. Clinical approval is likely to substantially catalyze the application of rTMS therapy, as well as research interest in this area.

16.7.1 Summary

rTMS shows considerable promise as a potential treatment for patients with a variety of addictive disorders. Deep TMS has recently been approved for use in smoking cessation although there is little accumulated clinical experience with this in real-world settings to date.

16.8 Chronic Pain

Due to the long-standing and often disabling nature of chronic pain, rTMS and other novel approaches using brain stimulation techniques have been investigated over a number of years. Approaches to the treatment of chronic pain with rTMS have focused on several different cortical sites. The main site for investigation, especially initially, has been the primary motor cortex. Studies since 2001 have utilized high- or low-frequency stimulation applied to the motor cortex to try to transiently or persistently ameliorate chronic pain. In the first study of this sort, investigators applied 10 Hz stimulation to the primary motor cortex of patients with intractable neurogenic pain. Pain relief was achieved with a single session of stimulation but this was short lasting and of modest effect [112]. A similar effect was seen in a second study investigating 10 Hz stimulation applied in patients with unilateral complex regional pain syndrome Type I of the hand [113].

Subsequent studies have explored longer periods of stimulation. For example, Picarelli et al. randomized 23 patients with complex regional pain syndrome Type 1 in the upper limb to commence standardized pharmacological treatment and either active or sham rTMS delivered in ten sessions at 10 Hz to the motor cortex contralateral to the affected side [114]. It was found that rTMS reduced pain intensities, particularly with ten treatment sessions, in a manner that was related to positive affective aspects of pain.

However, the analgesic effects of rTMS have not been consistent across studies with a number of negative studies reported (see review in [115]). Low-frequency rTMS appears to be less effective than high-frequency rTMS [116], and response appears to be dependent on the type of pain syndrome with facial pain, especially trigeminal neuralgia, appearing to respond better than other types of pain syndromes

[115]. A Cochrane review which included 19 rTMS studies concluded that there was evidence for short-term analgesic effects of single rTMS sessions, but limited evidence at this stage of longer-term treatment benefit [116]. Several other more recent reviews have concluded that analgesic effects are produced with both single rTMS sessions and longer durations of treatment but these effects are modest and require significantly more substantial studies to establish the role of this form of stimulation in clinical treatment [117, 118].

A second site for potential treatment of chronic pain with rTMS is the dorsolateral prefrontal cortex (DLPFC) due to its role in top-down modulation of pain. Tolerability of experimentally induced pain has been shown to be modulated both by high-frequency stimulation of the left DLPFC [119] and by low-frequency stimulation of the right DLPFC [120], both antidepressant rTMS paradigms. Early studies have begun to explore the potential of this form of stimulation in patients with chronic pain. For example, Borckardt et al. found analgesic effects of high-frequency left DLPFC stimulation in a small group of patients with neuropathic pain [121] and studies have also explored the potential benefits of high-frequency left DLPFC rTMS in distributed pain syndromes such as fibromyalgia [122–124]. In contrast, 1 Hz stimulation applied to the right DLPFC may produce benefit in patients with pain related to fibromyalgia [125].

16.8.1 Summary

Promising initial research suggests that rTMS may be able to modulate chronic pain when applied to either motor cortex or prefrontal brain regions depending on clinical application. However, the diversity of studies conducted to date make this literature difficult to interpret, and a lack of consistent studies using a single stimulation paradigm in one pain syndrome has stifled clinical translation.

References

1. Daskalakis ZJ et al (2006) The effects of repetitive transcranial magnetic stimulation on cortical inhibition in healthy human subjects. Exp Brain Res 174(3):403–412
2. Lefaucheur JP et al (2006) Motor cortex rTMS restores defective intracortical inhibition in chronic neuropathic pain. Neurology 67(9):1568–1574
3. Huang YZ et al (2008) Effect of physiological activity on an NMDA-dependent form of cortical plasticity in human. Cereb Cortex 18(3):563–570
4. Zai G et al (2005) Evidence for the gamma-amino-butyric acid type B receptor 1 (GABBR1) gene as a susceptibility factor in obsessive-compulsive disorder. Am J Med Genet B Neuropsychiatr Genet 134B(1):25–29
5. Arnold PD et al (2006) Glutamate transporter gene SLC1A1 associated with obsessive-compulsive disorder. Arch Gen Psychiatry 63(7):769–776
6. Greenberg BD et al (1997) Effects of single treatment with rTMS at different brain sites in depression. Electroencephalogr Clin Neurophysiol 103:A77
7. Sachdev PS et al (2007) Repetitive transcranial magnetic stimulation for the treatment of obsessive compulsive disorder: a double-blind controlled investigation. Psychol Med 37(11):1645–1649

8. Sarkhel S, Sinha VK, Praharaj SK (2010) Adjunctive high-frequency right prefrontal repetitive transcranial magnetic stimulation (rTMS) was not effective in obsessive-compulsive disorder but improved secondary depression. J Anxiety Disord 24(5):535–539
9. Alonso P et al (2001) Right prefrontal repetitive transcranial magnetic stimulation in obsessive-compulsive disorder: a double-blind, placebo-controlled study. Am J Psychiatry 158(7):1143–1145
10. Prasko J et al (2006) The effect of repetitive transcranial magnetic stimulation (rTMS) on symptoms in obsessive compulsive disorder. A randomized, double blind, sham controlled study. Neuro Endocrinol Lett 27(3):327–332
11. Seo HJ et al (2016) Adjunctive low-frequency repetitive transcranial magnetic stimulation over the right dorsolateral prefrontal cortex in patients with treatment-resistant obsessive-compulsive disorder: a randomized controlled trial. Clin Psychopharmacol Neurosci 14(2):153–160
12. Mantovani A et al (2006) Repetitive transcranial magnetic stimulation (rTMS) in the treatment of obsessive-compulsive disorder (OCD) and Tourette's syndrome (TS). Int J Neuropsychopharmacol 9(1):95–100
13. Mantovani A et al (2010) Randomized sham-controlled trial of repetitive transcranial magnetic stimulation in treatment-resistant obsessive-compulsive disorder. Int J Neuropsychopharmacol 13(2):217–227
14. Kang JI et al (2009) A randomized controlled study of sequentially applied repetitive transcranial magnetic stimulation in obsessive-compulsive disorder. J Clin Psychiatry 70(12):1645–1651
15. Lee YJ et al (2017) Repetitive transcranial magnetic stimulation of the supplementary motor area in treatment-resistant obsessive-compulsive disorder: an open-label pilot study. J Clin Neurosci 44:264–268
16. Pallanti S et al (2016) Better than treated as usual: transcranial magnetic stimulation augmentation in selective serotonin reuptake inhibitor-refractory obsessive-compulsive disorder, mini-review and pilot open-label trial. J Psychopharmacol 30(6):568–578
17. Pelissolo A et al (2016) Repetitive transcranial magnetic stimulation to supplementary motor area in refractory obsessive-compulsive disorder treatment: a sham-controlled trial. Int J Neuropsychopharmacol 19(8):pyw025
18. Ruffini C et al (2009) Augmentation effect of repetitive transcranial magnetic stimulation over the orbitofrontal cortex in drug-resistant obsessive-compulsive disorder patients: a controlled investigation. Prim Care Companion J Clin Psychiatry 11(5):226–230
19. Nauczyciel C et al (2014) Repetitive transcranial magnetic stimulation over the orbitofrontal cortex for obsessive-compulsive disorder: a double-blind, crossover study. Transl Psychiatry 4:e436
20. Carmi L et al (2019) Efficacy and safety of deep transcranial magnetic stimulation for obsessive-compulsive disorder: a prospective multicenter randomized double-blind placebo-controlled trial. Am J Psychiatry 176(11):931–938
21. Roth Y et al (2021) Real-world efficacy of deep TMS for obsessive-compulsive disorder: post-marketing data collected from twenty-two clinical sites. J Psychiatr Res 137:667–672
22. Perera MPN et al (2021) Repetitive transcranial magnetic stimulation (rTMS) for obsessive compulsive disorder (OCD): a meta-analysis of randomised, sham-controlled trials. Biol Psychiatry Cogn Neurosci Neuroimaging 6(10):947–960
23. Liang K et al (2021) Efficacy and tolerability of repetitive transcranial magnetic stimulation for the treatment of obsessive-compulsive disorder in adults: a systematic review and network meta-analysis. Transl Psychiatry 11(1):332
24. Grisaru N et al (1998) Transcranial magnetic stimulation in mania: a controlled study. Am J Psychiatry 155(11):1608–1610
25. Michael N, Erfurth A (2004) Treatment of bipolar mania with right prefrontal rapid transcranial magnetic stimulation. J Affect Disord 78(3):253–257
26. Saba G et al (2004) Repetitive transcranial magnetic stimulation as an add-on therapy in the treatment of mania: a case series of eight patients. Psychiatry Res 128(2):199–202

27. Kaptsan A et al (2003) Right prefrontal TMS versus sham treatment of mania: a controlled study. Bipolar Disord 5(1):36–39
28. Praharaj SK, Ram D, Arora M (2009) Efficacy of high frequency (rapid) suprathreshold repetitive transcranial magnetic stimulation of right prefrontal cortex in bipolar mania: a randomized sham controlled study. J Affect Disord 117(3):146–150
29. Grisaru N et al (1998) Effect of transcranial magnetic stimulation in posttraumatic stress disorder: a preliminary study. Biol Psychiatry 44(1):52–55
30. Rosenberg PB et al (2002) Repetitive transcranial magnetic stimulation treatment of comorbid posttraumatic stress disorder and major depression. J Neuropsychiatry Clin Neurosci 14(3):270–276
31. Cohen H et al (2004) Repetitive transcranial magnetic stimulation of the right dorsolateral prefrontal cortex in posttraumatic stress disorder: a double-blind, placebo-controlled study. Am J Psychiatry 161(3):515–524
32. Boggio PS et al (2010) Noninvasive brain stimulation with high-frequency and low-intensity repetitive transcranial magnetic stimulation treatment for posttraumatic stress disorder. J Clin Psychiatry 71(8):992–999
33. Watts BV et al (2012) A sham controlled study of repetitive transcranial magnetic stimulation for posttraumatic stress disorder. Brain Stimul 5(1):38–43
34. Paes F et al (2011) The value of repetitive transcranial magnetic stimulation (rTMS) for the treatment of anxiety disorders: an integrative review. CNS Neurol Disord Drug Targets 10(5):610–620
35. Isserles M et al (2013) Effectiveness of deep transcranial magnetic stimulation combined with a brief exposure procedure in post-traumatic stress disorder—a pilot study. Brain Stimul 6(3):377–383
36. Kozel FA et al (2018) Repetitive TMS to augment cognitive processing therapy in combat veterans of recent conflicts with PTSD: a randomized clinical trial. J Affect Disord 229:506–514
37. Kan RLD et al (2020) Non-invasive brain stimulation for posttraumatic stress disorder: a systematic review and meta-analysis. Transl Psychiatry 10(1):168
38. Prasko J et al (2007) The effect of repetitive transcranial magnetic stimulation (rTMS) add on serotonin reuptake inhibitors in patients with panic disorder: a randomized, double blind sham controlled study. Neuro Endocrinol Lett 28(1):33–38
39. Mantovani A et al (2013) Randomized sham controlled trial of repetitive transcranial magnetic stimulation to the dorsolateral prefrontal cortex for the treatment of panic disorder with comorbid major depression. J Affect Disord 144(1–2):153–159
40. Bystritsky A et al (2008) A preliminary study of fMRI-guided rTMS in the treatment of generalized anxiety disorder. J Clin Psychiatry 69(7):1092–1098
41. Diefenbach GJ et al (2016) Repetitive transcranial magnetic stimulation for generalised anxiety disorder: a pilot randomised, double-blind, sham-controlled trial. Br J Psychiatry 209(3):222–228
42. Chen L et al (2019) Is rTMS effective for anxiety symptoms in major depressive disorder? An efficacy analysis comparing left-sided high-frequency, right-sided low-frequency, and sequential bilateral rTMS protocols. Depress Anxiety 36(8):723–731
43. Paes F et al (2013) rTMS to treat social anxiety disorder: a case report. Rev Bras Psiquiatr 35(1):99–100
44. Paes F et al (2013) Repetitive transcranial magnetic stimulation (rTMS) to treat social anxiety disorder: case reports and a review of the literature. Clin Pract Epidemiol Ment Health 9:180–188
45. Lieberman JA et al (2005) Effectiveness of antipsychotic drugs in patients with chronic schizophrenia. N Engl J Med 353(12):1209–1223
46. Andreasen NC et al (1997) Hypofrontality in schizophrenia: distributed dysfunctional circuits in neuroleptic-naive patients. Lancet 349(9067):1730–1734
47. Cohen E et al (1999) Repetitive transcranial magnetic stimulation in the treatment of chronic negative schizophrenia: a pilot study. J Neurol Neurosurg Psychiatry 67(1):129–130

48. Shergill SS et al (2000) Mapping auditory hallucinations in schizophrenia using functional magnetic resonance imaging. Arch Gen Psychiatry 57(11):1033–1038
49. Silbersweig DA et al (1995) A functional neuroanatomy of hallucinations in schizophrenia. Nature 378(6553):176–179
50. Hoffman RE et al (1999) Transcranial magnetic stimulation of left temporoparietal cortex in three patients reporting hallucinated "voices". Biol Psychiatry 46(1):130–132
51. Hoffman RE et al (2000) Transcranial magnetic stimulation and auditory hallucinations in schizophrenia. Lancet 355(9209):1073–1075
52. Geller V et al (1997) Slow magnetic stimulation of prefrontal cortex in depression and schizophrenia. Prog Neuropsychopharmacol Biol Psychiatry 21(1):105–110
53. Feinsod M et al (1998) Preliminary evidence for a beneficial effect of low-frequency, repetitive transcranial magnetic stimulation in patients with major depression and schizophrenia. Depress Anxiety 7(2):65–68
54. Klein E et al (1999) Right prefrontal slow repetitive transcranial magnetic stimulation in schizophrenia: a double-blind sham-controlled pilot study. Biol Psychiatry 46(10):1451–1454
55. Rollnik JD et al (2000) High frequency repetitive transcranial magnetic stimulation (rTMS) of the dorsolateral prefrontal cortex in schizophrenic patients. Neuroreport 11(18):4013–4015
56. Holi MM et al (2004) Left prefrontal repetitive transcranial magnetic stimulation in schizophrenia. Schizophr Bull 30(2):429–434
57. Sachdev P et al (2005) Transcranial magnetic stimulation for the deficit syndrome of schizophrenia: a pilot investigation. Psychiatry Clin Neurosci 59(3):354–357
58. Hajak G et al (2004) High-frequency repetitive transcranial magnetic stimulation in schizophrenia: a combined treatment and neuroimaging study. Psychol Med 34(7):1157–1163
59. Freitas C, Fregni F, Pascual-Leone A (2009) Meta-analysis of the effects of repetitive transcranial magnetic stimulation (rTMS) on negative and positive symptoms in schizophrenia. Schizophr Res 108(1–3):11–24
60. Mogg A et al (2007) Repetitive transcranial magnetic stimulation for negative symptoms of schizophrenia: a randomized controlled pilot study. Schizophr Res 93(1–3):221–228
61. Novak T et al (2006) The double-blind sham-controlled study of high-frequency rTMS (20 Hz) for negative symptoms in schizophrenia: negative results. Neuro Endocrinol Lett 27(1–2):209–213
62. Prikryl R et al (2007) Treatment of negative symptoms of schizophrenia using repetitive transcranial magnetic stimulation in a double-blind, randomized controlled study. Schizophr Res 95(1–3):151–157
63. Jandl M et al (2005) Changes in negative symptoms and EEG in schizophrenic patients after repetitive transcranial magnetic stimulation (rTMS): an open-label pilot study. J Neural Transm 112(7):955–967
64. Goyal N, Nizamie SH, Desarkar P (2007) Efficacy of adjuvant high frequency repetitive transcranial magnetic stimulation on negative and positive symptoms of schizophrenia: preliminary results of a double-blind sham-controlled study. J Neuropsychiatry Clin Neurosci 19(4):464–467
65. Jin Y et al (2006) Therapeutic effects of individualized alpha frequency transcranial magnetic stimulation (alphaTMS) on the negative symptoms of schizophrenia. Schizophr Bull 32(3):556–561
66. Barr MS et al (2012) A randomized controlled trial of sequentially bilateral prefrontal cortex repetitive transcranial magnetic stimulation in the treatment of negative symptoms in schizophrenia. Brain Stimul 5(3):337–346
67. Fitzgerald PB et al (2008) A study of the effectiveness of bilateral transcranial magnetic stimulation in the treatment of the negative symptoms of schizophrenia. Brain Stimul 1(1):27–32
68. Wobrock T et al (2015) Left prefrontal high-frequency repetitive transcranial magnetic stimulation for the treatment of schizophrenia with predominant negative symptoms: a sham-controlled, randomized multicenter trial. Biol Psychiatry 77(11):979–988

69. Quan WX et al (2015) The effects of high-frequency repetitive transcranial magnetic stimulation (rTMS) on negative symptoms of schizophrenia and the follow-up study. Neurosci Lett 584:197–201
70. Dlabac-de Lange JJ et al (2015) Efficacy of bilateral repetitive transcranial magnetic stimulation for negative symptoms of schizophrenia: results of a multicenter double-blind randomized controlled trial. Psychol Med 45(6):1263–1275
71. Zhao S et al (2014) Randomized controlled trial of four protocols of repetitive transcranial magnetic stimulation for treating the negative symptoms of schizophrenia. Shanghai Arch Psychiatry 26(1):15–21
72. Aleman A et al (2018) Moderate effects of noninvasive brain stimulation of the frontal cortex for improving negative symptoms in schizophrenia: meta-analysis of controlled trials. Neurosci Biobehav Rev 89:111–118
73. Osoegawa C et al (2018) Non-invasive brain stimulation for negative symptoms in schizophrenia: an updated systematic review and meta-analysis. Schizophr Res 197:34–44
74. Heinrichs RW (2005) The primacy of cognition in schizophrenia. Am Psychol 60(3):229–242
75. Barr MS et al (2009) Potentiation of gamma oscillatory activity through repetitive transcranial magnetic stimulation of the dorsolateral prefrontal cortex. Neuropsychopharmacology 34(11):2359–2367
76. Barr MS et al (2011) The effect of repetitive transcranial magnetic stimulation on gamma oscillatory activity in schizophrenia. PLoS One 6(7):e22627
77. Guse B et al (2013) The effect of long-term high frequency repetitive transcranial magnetic stimulation on working memory in schizophrenia and healthy controls—a randomized placebo-controlled, double-blind fMRI study. Behav Brain Res 237:300–307
78. Zhuo K et al (2019) Repetitive transcranial magnetic stimulation as an adjunctive treatment for negative symptoms and cognitive impairment in patients with schizophrenia: a randomized, double-blind, sham-controlled trial. Neuropsychiatr Dis Treat 15:1141–1150
79. Jiang Y et al (2019) Effects of high-frequency transcranial magnetic stimulation for cognitive deficit in schizophrenia: a meta-analysis. Front Psychiatry 10:135
80. Hoffman RE et al (2003) Transcranial magnetic stimulation of left temporoparietal cortex and medication-resistant auditory hallucinations. Arch Gen Psychiatry 60(1):49–56
81. Hoffman RE et al (2005) Temporoparietal transcranial magnetic stimulation for auditory hallucinations: safety, efficacy and moderators in a fifty patient sample. Biol Psychiatry 58(2):97–104
82. Brunelin J et al (2006) Low frequency repetitive transcranial magnetic stimulation improves source monitoring deficit in hallucinating patients with schizophrenia. Schizophr Res 81(1):41–45
83. Chibbaro G et al (2005) Repetitive transcranial magnetic stimulation in schizophrenic patients reporting auditory hallucinations. Neurosci Lett 383(1–2):54–57
84. d'Alfonso AA et al (2002) Transcranial magnetic stimulation of left auditory cortex in patients with schizophrenia: effects on hallucinations and neurocognition. J Neuropsychiatry Clin Neurosci 14(1):77–79
85. Fitzgerald PB et al (2005) A double-blind sham-controlled trial of repetitive transcranial magnetic stimulation in the treatment of refractory auditory hallucinations. J Clin Psychopharmacol 25(4):358–362
86. Jandl M et al (2006) Treating auditory hallucinations by transcranial magnetic stimulation: a randomized controlled cross-over trial. Neuropsychobiology 53(2):63–69
87. McIntosh AM et al (2004) Transcranial magnetic stimulation for auditory hallucinations in schizophrenia. Psychiatry Res 127(1–2):9–17
88. Poulet E et al (2005) Slow transcranial magnetic stimulation can rapidly reduce resistant auditory hallucinations in schizophrenia. Biol Psychiatry 57(2):188–191
89. Saba G, Schurhoff F, Leboyer M (2006) Therapeutic and neurophysiologic aspects of transcranial magnetic stimulation in schizophrenia. Neurophysiol Clin 36(3):185–194

90. Horacek J et al (2007) Effect of low-frequency rTMS on electromagnetic tomography (LORETA) and regional brain metabolism (PET) in schizophrenia patients with auditory hallucinations. Neuropsychobiology 55(3–4):132–142
91. Bagati D, Nizamie SH, Prakash R (2009) Effect of augmentatory repetitive transcranial magnetic stimulation on auditory hallucinations in schizophrenia: randomized controlled study. Aust N Z J Psychiatry 43(4):386–392
92. Vercammen A et al (2009) Effects of bilateral repetitive transcranial magnetic stimulation on treatment resistant auditory-verbal hallucinations in schizophrenia: a randomized controlled trial. Schizophr Res 114(1–3):172–179
93. Rosa MO et al (2007) Effects of repetitive transcranial magnetic stimulation on auditory hallucinations refractory to clozapine. J Clin Psychiatry 68(10):1528–1532
94. Aleman A, Sommer IE, Kahn RS (2007) Efficacy of slow repetitive transcranial magnetic stimulation in the treatment of resistant auditory hallucinations in schizophrenia: a meta-analysis. J Clin Psychiatry 68(3):416–421
95. Slotema CW et al (2014) Review of the efficacy of transcranial magnetic stimulation for auditory verbal hallucinations. Biol Psychiatry 76(2):101–110
96. Otani VH et al (2014) A systematic review and meta-analysis of the use of repetitive transcranial magnetic stimulation for auditory hallucinations treatment in refractory schizophrenic patients. Int J Psychiatry Clin Pract 19(4):228–232
97. Slotema CW et al (2010) Should we expand the toolbox of psychiatric treatment methods to include repetitive transcranial magnetic stimulation (rTMS)? A meta-analysis of the efficacy of rTMS in psychiatric disorders. J Clin Psychiatry 71(7):873–884
98. He H et al (2017) Repetitive transcranial magnetic stimulation for treating the symptoms of schizophrenia: a PRISMA compliant meta-analysis. Clin Neurophysiol 128(5):716–724
99. Kennedy NI, Lee WH, Frangou S (2018) Efficacy of non-invasive brain stimulation on the symptom dimensions of schizophrenia: a meta-analysis of randomized controlled trials. Eur Psychiatry 49:69–77
100. Schonfeldt-Lecuona C et al (2004) Stereotaxic rTMS for the treatment of auditory hallucinations in schizophrenia. Neuroreport 15(10):1669–1673
101. Sommer IE et al (2007) Can fMRI-guidance improve the efficacy of rTMS treatment for auditory verbal hallucinations? Schizophr Res 93(1–3):406–408
102. Hoffman RE et al (2007) Probing the pathophysiology of auditory/verbal hallucinations by combining functional magnetic resonance imaging and transcranial magnetic stimulation. Cereb Cortex 17(11):2733–2743
103. Dollfus S et al (2008) Treatment of auditory hallucinations by combining high-frequency repetitive transcranial magnetic stimulation and functional magnetic resonance imaging. Schizophr Res 102(1–3):348–351
104. Pascual-Leone A, Gates JR, Dhuna A (1991) Induction of speech arrest and counting errors with rapid-rate transcranial magnetic stimulation. Neurology 41(5):697–702
105. Montagne-Larmurier A et al (2009) Two-day treatment of auditory hallucinations by high frequency rTMS guided by cerebral imaging: a 6 month follow-up pilot study. Schizophr Res 113(1):77–83
106. Fitzgerald PB et al (2006) The treatment of recurring auditory hallucinations in schizophrenia with rTMS. World J Biol Psychiatry 7(2):119–122
107. Poulet E et al (2006) Is rTMS efficient as a maintenance treatment for auditory verbal hallucinations? A case report. Schizophr Res 84(1):183–184
108. Thirthalli J et al (2008) Successful use of maintenance rTMS for 8 months in a patient with antipsychotic-refractory auditory hallucinations. Schizophr Res 100(1–3):351–352
109. Poulet E et al (2008) Maintenance treatment with transcranial magnetic stimulation in a patient with late-onset schizophrenia. Am J Psychiatry 165(4):537–538
110. Hanlon CA, Dowdle LT, Henderson JS (2018) Modulating neural circuits with transcranial magnetic stimulation: implications for addiction treatment development. Pharmacol Rev 70(3):661–683

111. Dinur-Klein L et al (2014) Smoking cessation induced by deep repetitive transcranial magnetic stimulation of the prefrontal and insular cortices: a prospective, randomized controlled trial. Biol Psychiatry 76(9):742–749
112. Lefaucheur JP et al (2001) Pain relief induced by repetitive transcranial magnetic stimulation of precentral cortex. Neuroreport 12(13):2963–2965
113. Pleger B et al (2004) Repetitive transcranial magnetic stimulation of the motor cortex attenuates pain perception in complex regional pain syndrome type I. Neurosci Lett 356(2):87–90
114. Picarelli H et al (2010) Repetitive transcranial magnetic stimulation is efficacious as an add-on to pharmacological therapy in complex regional pain syndrome (CRPS) type I. J Pain 11(11):1203–1210
115. Plow EB, Pascual-Leone A, Machado A (2012) Brain stimulation in the treatment of chronic neuropathic and non-cancerous pain. J Pain 13(5):411–424
116. O'Connell NE et al (2011) Non-invasive brain stimulation techniques for chronic pain. A report of a Cochrane systematic review and meta-analysis. Eur J Phys Rehabil Med 47(2):309–326
117. Gatzinsky K et al (2020) Repetitive transcranial magnetic stimulation of the primary motor cortex in management of chronic neuropathic pain: a systematic review. Scand J Pain 21(1):8–21
118. Hamid P, Malik BH, Hussain ML (2019) Noninvasive transcranial magnetic stimulation (TMS) in chronic refractory pain: a systematic review. Cureus 11(10):e6019
119. Borckardt JJ et al (2007) Fifteen minutes of left prefrontal repetitive transcranial magnetic stimulation acutely increases thermal pain thresholds in healthy adults. Pain Res Manag 12(4):287–290
120. Graff-Guerrero A et al (2005) Repetitive transcranial magnetic stimulation of dorsolateral prefrontal cortex increases tolerance to human experimental pain. Brain Res Cogn Brain Res 25(1):153–160
121. Borckardt JJ et al (2009) A pilot study investigating the effects of fast left prefrontal rTMS on chronic neuropathic pain. Pain Med 10(5):840–849
122. Short EB et al (2011) Ten sessions of adjunctive left prefrontal rTMS significantly reduces fibromyalgia pain: a randomized, controlled pilot study. Pain 152(11):2477–2484
123. Fitzgibbon BM et al (2018) Evidence for the improvement of fatigue in fibromyalgia: a 4-week left dorsolateral prefrontal cortex repetitive transcranial magnetic stimulation randomized-controlled trial. Eur J Pain 22(7):1255–1267
124. Bilir I et al (2021) Effects of high frequency neuronavigated repetitive transcranial magnetic stimulation in fibromyalgia syndrome: a double-blinded, randomized controlled study. Am J Phys Med Rehabil 100(2):138–146
125. Sampson SM et al (2011) The use of slow-frequency prefrontal repetitive transcranial magnetic stimulation in refractory neuropathic pain. J ECT 27(1):33–37

Equipment and rTMS Program Setup 17

Abstract

There are multiple manufacturers of devices that may be utilized in the rTMS treatment of depression and other disorders. However, the characteristics of the equipment produced by each manufacturer vary considerably. Prior to purchase of equipment, a variety of factors should be considered, including the stimulation parameters able to be provided, whether coil cooling is an issue, and local regulatory status. In the establishment of a clinical rTMS service, a variety of factors should be resolved prior to commencement of treatment. Procedures should be in place to manage the intake and assessment of patients and their management during rTMS treatment and during follow-up. Adequate provision needs to be made to ensure that patients provide sufficiently informed consent.

17.1 TMS Equipment

There are currently a progressively increasing number of TMS equipment manufacturers. However, the accessibility of equipment for the provision of rTMS treatment will vary greatly country by country, limited by local regulatory approval and the availability of local distribution.

Beyond these obvious practical issues, a number of factors should be taken into account when selecting TMS equipment for clinical application. One of the most important is the capacity of stimulators to provide stimulation in the manner required for particular treatment protocols. There is variation across stimulation devices in the ranges of frequencies and intensities able to be provided, especially at stimulation frequencies greater than 20 Hz which are likely to be most relevant when considering the potential use of novel paradigms such as theta-burst stimulation (TBS).

A common and critical consideration is whether the coil being utilized for stimulation will provide an adequate number of pulses without overheating. There is

P. B. Fitzgerald, Z. J. Daskalakis, *rTMS Treatment for Depression*,
https://doi.org/10.1007/978-3-030-91519-3_17

considerable variation in the systems used to provide long periods of stimulation without coil overheating across device manufacturers. These include the development of iron core coils and the integration of fluid cooling systems and fan-based cooling systems. Prior to the selection of a stimulator and coil, potential users should ensure that a sufficient number of pulses at high intensity can be provided for each individual treatment session, but also that individual treatment sessions can be provided consecutively with only short between patient intervals if required. It is highly likely that some systems may able to operate throughout an individual treatment, but if multiple treatments are being provided rapidly back to back, this can become an issue with some, typically older, coil systems.

It is also important to confirm that the system is provided with adequate accessories to ensure the smooth operation of treatment sessions. Coil stands and localization positioning systems vary substantially across equipment manufacturers and should be evaluated prior to equipment purchase. The software system to control stimulation protocols should also be evaluated: these are progressively improving but some systems are not very end user-friendly. The best systems currently available tend to have the capacity to predetermine a set of protocols which can be selected for each individual patient so that individual elements of treatment such as frequency, train duration, etc. do not need to be individually entered. Some systems will also have the capacity to store medical record-related information although most clinics will not require this in addition to the operation of the TMS equipment itself.

A final but critical consideration is the availability of timely onsite equipment support. rTMS equipment is technically complex and utilizes high electrical voltages. As such, equipment malfunction should be expected to occur occasionally and local technical staff may not be qualified to service and repair equipment. As most equipment is quite heavy and bulky, shipping back to a device manufacturer for repair can be expensive, slow, and problematic. In establishing a clinical service, thought may be given to ensuring the availability of backup equipment to prevent the interruption of clinical programs should equipment fail. It seems sensible and financially viable to ensure the local availability of backup coils; however, resourcing local backup stimulators may well be more problematic. The purchase and storage of some backup coils can be problematic if there is a lifespan on usage. Questions should be asked of distributors as to whether replacement devices on loan are available during equipment repair.

The following is a brief description of a number of currently available TMS devices and manufacturers.

17.2 MagVenture

MagPro TMS stimulators have been produced since the early 1990s by Tonica Elektronik in Denmark and, over time, sold under the brands of Dantec, Medtronic, and currently MagVenture. Several MagPro devices are currently available, servicing both clinical and research TMS communities. For the treatment of depression, the most commonly utilized devices are likely to be the MagPro R30 and the MagPro R100. These machines are very similar in design and utilize the same stimulation coils. The main difference is the frequency/intensity at which stimulation can be provided: the MagPro R30 is effectively limited to below 30 Hz, while the MagPro R100 can provide stimulation at up to 100 Hz. In the routine treatment of depression utilizing protocols in the 1–20 Hz range, this difference is insignificant and a MagPro R30 is likely to suffice. If there is a need for more experimental protocols, for example, considering TBS and higher stimulation intensities, a R100 device may be considered appropriate although there are upgrades to the MagPro R30 that allow the use of TBS.

The MagPro R30 device is relatively compact and is sold with optional accessories including a coil stand, stimulator trolley, and device for displaying EMG data during the assessment of resting motor thresholds. There are a number of coils available. The most useful coil for clinical applications is a "dynamically" cooled figure-of-eight coil, which is sold with a separate fluid-based cooling system. Of note, MagVenture have a double cone coil available which has been FDA approved for the treatment of obsessive-compulsive disorder. This can be relatively easily exchanged with the standard figure-of-eight coil used in depression treatment between patients although the front plate of the cooling system needs to be removed with a screwdriver to do this, and is then probably sensibly left off if coils are being changed frequently.

More recently MagVenture have been marketing and selling what is described as their MagVenture TMS therapy system. This comprises the stimulator itself, a TMS coil for motor threshold determination, the treatment coil, the cooling system, a trolley and coil stand, a custom-built treatment chair, and a pillow designed to shape around the head keeping the head still during treatment. Cotton caps are available to facilitate the marking of the patient's location.

In our experience, these devices allow the application of long stimulation protocols without any substantial coil overheating during or between closely spaced patient sessions. The MagPro systems are widely available in North America, Europe, and other countries including Australia.

17.3 Magstim

Magstim has also been selling TMS systems for many years for a variety of research and clinical applications and dates back to the initial discovery of the use of TMS in Sheffield in the UK. There are multiple Magstim systems available that are suitable for clinical use. Historically these have included the Magstim Rapid[2], the Super Rapid, and Super Rapid Plus. These three units essentially vary only in the stimulation frequencies and intensities that are able to be applied during stimulation protocols. A choice between these devices, like the choice between the MagPro R30 and R100, will be predominately driven by user needs. A series of different coil types are available for the Magstim systems. These include a cooled coil using a fan mounted close to the coil itself. Coil stands and other accessories are also available.

Magstim is also now offering their system in a series of packages they refer to as Magstim TMS therapy. This includes the Horizon Lite and the Horizon Performance along with an optional neuronavigational option. The Horizon Lite system includes a basic simulator, chair, coil stand, and air film cooled coil. The Horizon Performance includes a high-powered simulator, a coil with more substantial cooling capacity, and a much more substantial coil support system to support the weight and complexity of this coil.

17.4 Neuronetics

Neuronetics is an American company that has developed and commercialized the NeuroStar TMS treatment system, which has been commercially available in the USA since 2008. The system was approved by the FDA for the treatment of major depressive disorder in patients who had failed to receive benefit from antidepressant therapy based on a large multisite trial conducted across a number of countries. The device is sold as an integrated system with stimulator, coil, coil positioning system, and software for assisting in estimation of the motor threshold. The commercial devices can only operate with a single use disposable "SenStar" device in place, which is proposed to ensure adequate coil functioning and localization. There is a significant cost for each of these devices, and they cannot be reused across treatment sessions even within an individual patient's course. The NeuroStar system has more recently been approved for use with a reduced intertrain interval (11 s) as well as TBS application.

17.5 Brainsway

Brainsway is an Israeli company that has commercialized a system for deep TMS (dTMS) using a series of Hesed or H-coils. In April 2012, the company announced positive results from a clinical trial evaluating dTMS treatment of 233 patients across 14 sites which subsequently led to FDA approval in the USA and many other countries around the world. dTMS for depression involves the use of the H1 coil which is provided with a simulator and cooling system. A separate H7 coil is available for the treatment of obsessive-compulsive disorder and the H4 for coil has been shown to be beneficial as an aid in short-term smoking cessation. Brainsway coils are also CE marked (not approved for use in the USA) for the treatment of bipolar disorder, PTSD, and schizophrenia.

17.6 Nexstim

Nexstim is a Finnish company that manufacturers TMS equipment developed and approved for use in neurosurgical planning as well as in the treatment of depression. The "SmartFocus TMS" system integrates neuronavigation with TMS treatment delivery in a manner which uses anatomical landmarks to localize a site of stimulation based on individual subject's MRI scans. The neuronavigational process has been set up in a way that is usable by clinicians with relatively limited degree of training in use of the specific system. The system comes with all of the standard accessories including a coil arm and holder, cooling, and a purpose-built reclining chair.

17.7 Neurosoft

Neurosoft is a Russian TMS manufacturer that produces the "CloudTMS" system which is relatively widely available and FDA approved in the USA. They have a range of configurations for their TMS equipment and multiple efficiently fluid cooled coils, again sold with a range of accessories for clinical treatment administration.

17.8 Others

There are an increasing number of other TMS equipment manufacturers making equipment available for clinical use in varying markets around the world. These include Mag & More (Germany), Deymed (Czech Republic), as well as a range of companies in Korea, India, and China.

17.9 Treatment Program Establishment

There are potentially a number of models for the provision of an rTMS clinical service and the appropriateness of these to local clinical and organizational needs should be considered. It is possible that rTMS could be provided within the office-based practice of an individual psychiatrist or a small group of clinicians. However, this type of approach may prove problematic if insufficient patients are regularly in treatment to justify the employment of an individual to actually provide treatment. Alternatively, rTMS treatment centers may be established on a local or regional basis, receiving referrals from a network of referring doctors and providing rTMS treatment only. This model may provide a more sensible concentration of expertise, but issues relating to the separation of rTMS from other forms of clinical care will need to be managed.

The setup of TMS programs will by necessity have to follow the local regulatory frameworks, including for the credentialing of rTMS clinic staff. Issues to be considered and clearly articulated include the establishment of referral pathways and processes for routine and emergency clinical review. The degree to which the provision of treatment with rTMS is integrated with the referred patient's overall treatment program is something that can be established on a patient-to-patient basis but should be at least in part determined by local policy. For example, when a patient is referred to a TMS clinical program, a clinician within the program, preferably a psychiatrist, will need to make ongoing decisions about TMS provision: for example, whether a sufficiently adequate course has been tried, should stimulation parameters change, when treatment should stop, and whether maintenance treatment should be considered.

However, simultaneously, decisions may need to be made in regard to altering other forms of treatment such as antidepressant or other medication. Regardless of whether these decisions are made by the rTMS program psychiatrist or the patient's original treating psychiatrist, communication is essential to ensure that problems don't eventuate. For example, motor threshold may need to be reassessed if medications are changed. In establishing a TMS program, thought should be given to establishing protocols to determine how these relationships are managed. In addition, it should be clear to the patient who is responsible for routine review of their mental state and for responding to psychiatric emergency such as an escalation of suicidal ideation.

In addition, formal protocols should be developed for emergency responses during rTMS provision. These will include a seizure response protocol and a protocol for response to other forms of loss of consciousness such as syncope. Documentation is required for the prescription of rTMS treatment and recording of all aspects of stimulation provided.

17.10 Patient Information and Consent

As with all significant medical procedures, patients should be provided with sufficient verbal and written information as to the nature of rTMS treatment, its risks, and its potential benefits to allow them to provide informed consent. This information should include a discussion of the likely efficacy of rTMS treatment, the potential risk of seizure induction, and the possibility of side effects such as treatment-related discomfort, pain, and headache. Patients should be informed in advance of the need to disclose any changes in medical status or medication treatment and drug or alcohol consumption during the course of rTMS therapy. Ideally they should also be informed as to the processes for emergency responses during the course of rTMS treatment and the roles of clinicians with whom they will have contact.

Index

P. B. Fitzgerald, Z. J. Daskalakis, *rTMS Treatment for Depression*,
https://doi.org/10.1007/978-3-030-91519-3

GPSR Compliance

The European Union's (EU) General Product Safety Regulation (GPSR) is a set of rules that requires consumer products to be safe and our obligations to ensure this.

If you have any concerns about our products, you can contact us on ProductSafety@springernature.com

In case Publisher is established outside the EU, the EU authorized representative is:

Springer Nature Customer Service Center GmbH
Europaplatz 3
69115 Heidelberg, Germany

Batch number: 10732044

Printed by Printforce, the Netherlands